YOUR VISION

"If you have any questions about your eyes, this book will give you the answers."
        -Charles D. Kelman, M.D.
        President-elect of American Society
        of Cataract and Refractive Surgery

"When I needed him, Dr. Cross was there with many simple, direct, and to-the-point explanations (about my eyes). I highly recommend *Your Vision* for anyone wishing to learn about eye problems and surgeries."
        -Lt. Gen. John R. Murphy, U.S.A.F. (RET.)
        Deputy Commander of United
        Nations Council and Commander
        of U.S. Forces, Korea

"Finally! An honest, informative guide through the maze of opthalmology for the lay person."
        -John Dew/Executive/Lansing, MI

"For me, good information and data are essential. *Your Vision* meets the criteria. An invaluable source!"
        -Jack A. Hewitt/V.P. T.R.W. Financial Systems
        Former Undersecretary, Dept. of Energy
        and Undersecretary, U.S. Air Force

"Dr. Cross patiently guides you through all of the aspects of eye care, diseases, the aging eye and surgeries which cure and correct. This book is interesting, informative and a must buy."
        -N. Daniel Moss, L.L.D./Chief Council/
        President of Frette linens, U.S.A.

"From eyeglasses and medicine to lasers and lens implants, this well-illustrated handbook proves invaluable for students, patients, and health care providers. I recommend *Your Vision* to all my patients."
        -John M. Corboy, M.D./Surgeon/
        Director, Hawaiian Eye Center
        Associate Clinical Professor, University
        of Hawaii School of Medicine

YOUR VISION

ALL ABOUT MODERN EYE CARE

Warren D. Cross, Jr., M.D.
Lawrence Lynn, Ph.D.

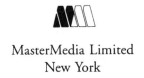

MasterMedia Limited
New York

Copyright © 1994 Warren D. Cross, Jr., and Lawrence Lynn.

Buying Glasses reprinted from *Consumer Reports*, August 1993.

We would like to give special thanks to Jan Redden, Medical Illustrator, Baylor College of Medicine, for her contribution to Your Vision: All About Modern Eye Care.

All rights reserved, including the right of reproduction in whole or in part in any form.

Published by MasterMedia Limited.

MASTERMEDIA and colophon are registered trademarks of MasterMedia Limited.

ISBN 1-57101-019-X (pbk.).

Production and design services by Martin Cook Associates, Ltd., New York.

Manufactured in the United States of America.

10 9 8 7 6 5 4 3 2 1

This book is dedicated to my grandmother, Carol Cross, who at age 96 will read this book with two "new eyes" as achieved by the procedures described herein; to America's future—our young people; to our "silver-haired" older generation from whom we have learned much, and who represent a yet untapped wealth and resource of knowledge, experience and energy; to our American system; to God, who created us; to my wife, Kathleen; to my children, Warren Cross III (Trey) and Melissa; and lastly, to my Doberman, Jazz, who slept at my feet.

—Warren D. Cross, M.D.

Contents

	Acknowledgments	ix
	Foreword	xi
	About the Authors	xiii
1	The Evolution of Eye Care	1
2	Anatomy and Physiology of the Eye	15
3	The Comprehensive Eye Examination	35
4	Refraction, Optics, and Eyeglasses	57
5	Cataracts and Their Treatment	73
6	Laser and Electromagnetic Energy and Eye Surgery	85
7	Glaucoma	93
8	Corneal Refractive Surgery	109
9	Diseases and Surgery of the Retina	129
10	Pediatric Eye Care	145
11	Corneal and External Disease	157
12	"Buying Glasses" Reprinted from *Consumer Reports*	187
13	Contact Lenses and Their Uses	213

14	Ophthalmic Plastic and Reconstructive Surgery	233
15	Visible Drug Effects	249
16	Ocular Emergencies	259
17	Understanding Insurance	269
18	Frequently Asked Questions	279
	Bibliography	295
	Index	299

Acknowledgments

We want to acknowledge the kind help from many people in the preparation of data and drawings, as well as the manuscript itself, for this book. A great debt of gratitude belongs to Jan Redden, Medical Illustrator of Baylor College of Medicine. We are also indebted to Alcon Pharmaceuticals, Neal J. Bailey, O.D., Bert Bandini, Robert C. Bockoven, M.D., David Brooks, David Castle, Steven H. Cobb, M.D., John M. Corboy, M.D., Carol Cross, Kathleen Cross, John Dew, George Dill, Karen Douglas, Bernard Friedman, M.D., Laura L. Garcia, O.D., Joseph S. Goetz, M.D., Karyn R. Hennessy, John A. Hewitt, Jr., Dick Hornback, Joseph Janes, O.D., Charles D. Kelman, M.D., Daniel Klaff, O.D., Dr. David Jolivet, Dan B. Jones, M.D., Professor and Chairman, Baylor College of Medicine, Houston, Evan D. Jones, M.D., Marianne Joy, Dr. Harvey Kornblit, Dr. Luis Lay, Jr., Dori Lynn, Robert Marmer, M.D., N. Daniel Moss, Donna O'Malley, Lt. Gen. John R. Murphy U.S.A.F. (ret.), George Stonewall Ormsby, Vivian Rodriguez, Ray Reyes, Robert H. Rubman, M.D., Linda Shepherd, O.D., Michael Suber, O.D., Richard Ruiz, M.D., Professor and Chairman, University of Texas Medical Branch, Houston, Jan and John Turley, and all the staff members at Bellaire Eye Associates and Institute of Eye Surgery for their help and encouragement in this project. Last and certainly not least, this work would not have been undertaken (and surely not finished!) without the suggestions and enthusiastic encouragement of many ophthalmological colleagues all over the country who realize how many patients frequently request a general book on ophthalmology written for the layman.

Finally, we want to acknowledge the valued help and encouragement provided by Michael Doran of Southern Literary Agency who also contributed in the editing and finalization of the manuscript.

Warren D. Cross, M.D.

Lawrence Lynn, Ph.D.

Foreword

Modern medicine uses increasingly sophisticated technologies to detect, diagnose and treat eye problems. The earlier you are aware of your symptoms, seek help and begin treatment, the more likely you are to circumvent catastrophic loss of vision. Care of your general physical health as well as avoidance of situations where you could seriously injure or damage your eyes increases your chances of maintaining good vision all of your life. It is our intent to educate and heighten your awareness of eye diseases and their prevention through this book, which we believe is destined to become your eye-care bible.

As medicine is changing, our country is becoming more conscious of prevention as opposed to treatment. Our chief goal is to satisfy your increasing demand for knowledge and self-education in relation to eye problems, their prevention, and treatment. This book empowers you with the ability to exercise preventative measures regarding eye care and furthermore the principles and thought processes described herein enable you to better select your physicians and choice of treatments for medical care—not just eye care. *Your Vision* will enable you to accurately verify alcohol and drug use in your children, friends, employees and essentially any individual suspected of drug use.

Today, virtually any eye problem can be treated. From the relatively crude tools of the ancient surgeons to our diamond knives and laser surgery today, this book offers the fascinating history of eye medicine and tells what can be done to produce the quality of vision our predecessors would have thought impossible. *Your Vision* appeals to basically all audiences: those with the interests of the informed layman, who are simply curious about a dynamic, burgeoning field of science; younger persons who have inherited vision problems or acquired them through accident and want to know what is available to treat them; the growing population of those who have lived long enough to develop the typical eye conditions of old age; and teachers, employers, and parents who long for a simple, accurate, quick and easy method of determining drug and alcohol use in those who may be under their influence. Every effort has been made to present information in the most interesting way, with a minimum of jargon but a good selection of illustrations, charts, and tables. Thus, while we are confident that the eye professional will find our narrative accurate and up-to-date, it has been written according to the needs of the great majority who will use it.

There has long been a need for *Your Vision: All About Modern Eye Care*. It is our hope that we have achieved a lasting contribution to the general public.

About the Authors

Dr. Warren D. Cross, co-author of this work, received his undergraduate education from the University of Southern California. As part of his undergraduate studies he attended Cambridge University in England. His formal medical education was at Baylor College of Medicine, Houston. He did his internship at The Methodist Hospital, Houston, followed by active duty as a U.S. Air Force flight surgeon. After serving as a flight surgeon, he held a residency with the University of Texas Medical Branch, Houston Ophthalmology Faculty. After training with Dr. Charles Kelman in New York, he was actively involved in cataract surgery courses. He served as an emergency room doctor in Houston and was a founder of Bellaire Eye Associates (BEA) in Houston. BEA is now one of the larger ophthalmic clinics in Texas. Dr. Cross currently serves as Medical Director and Chief Surgeon. He has published several books and articles on refractive surgery.

Dr. Lawrence Lynn did his undergraduate and graduate work at Texas A&M and Columbia University in engineering. He has published many scientific and economic papers in the fields of chemical and food technology.

Upon finishing his education, Dr. Lynn returned to Texas to work in research and engineering. After moving into management, he was elected President and CEO of Pine-O-Pine, a household chemical-specialties manufacturer, headquartered in Houston. He entered the brokerage-investment banking community in Houston, beginning with Merrill Lynch, and later serving as Senior Vice-President at Drexel Burnham Lambert. Since 1984, he has been teaching (part-time) adult classes in investments, and he is the editor of the new investment guide *How to Invest Today*. He lives in Houston now with his wife, two dogs, and a cat.

Dr. Lynn became a cataract patient in mid-1990, when his eyesight in both eyes was restored from 20/200 (legally blind) to 20/25 by a colleague of Dr. Cross.

Keith A. Bourgeois, M.D., studied zoology as an undergraduate, then medicine afterwards, receiving his degrees from Louisiana State University. Interning in Lafayette, Louisiana, at University Medical Center, he holds a post-resident fellowship in vitroretinal studies at the Hermann Eye Center in Houston. Presently, Dr. Bourgeois is an instructor at the University of Texas Health Science Center and a staff member of Bellaire Eye Associates in Houston, Texas. He is the contributor of Chapter Nine: Diseases and Surgery of the Retina.

Stacey L. Brown, C.O.A. (Certified Ophthalmic Assistant), has a background of six years of extensive ophthalmological training. She attended college in East Texas, majoring in Graphic Arts, Communications and Photography, after which she attained her C.O.A. She has participated in the publication of numerous ophthalmological manuscripts and is currently involved in the initial investigational phase of the Schachar Scleral Expander Band, a surgical procedure for the correction of presbyopia. She is currently Executive Secretary of the Institute of Eye Surgery and has contributed to Chapter Three: The Comprehensive Eye Examination.

Joseph H. Fitzgerald is an independent consultant on medical office management and claims-filing techniques for nearly a hundred clinics in the United States. He has a B.B.A. from the University of Dallas and has served as business and administrative manager for chains of hospitals in California. He has contributed to Chapter Seventeen: Understanding Insurance.

Jim Pietrantonio, O.D., is the contributor of Chapter Thirteen: Contact Lenses. He attended San Jose State University as an undergraduate and the University of Houston for his studies in optometry. Dr. Pietrantonio, formerly the Clinical Director at Bellaire Eye Associates, supervised the intern education for optometry students on the staff.

About the Authors

Pamela Pullings has contributed to Chapter Seventeen: Understanding Insurance. She trained through the Technical Institute for Ophthalmology Management and Senior Technicians in 1984 in Boston, Mass. She is currently the Business Office Manager for a leading clinic in Houston, Texas, as well as the Manager for Billing and Insurance of the Institute of Eye Surgery, Houston. She is active in the American Society of Ophthalmic Administrators and consults with other physicians' staff in cost-effective methods of billing and collections.

Martha C. Wilson, M.D., an undergraduate at the National University of Mexico and Louisiana State, received her M.D. from the University of Louisville. She did her residency at Duke Eye Center in Durham, N.C., and served as a fellow at the Jules Stein Eye Institute at U.C.L.A. She has served as a reconstructive ophthalmic surgeon since then in San Antonio and Houston, Texas, and is the author of many papers on adult and pediatric epidemiology. Dr. Wilson's frequent Spanish-language television appearances are most popular and are frequently aired from Mexico to Argentina. She is one of the most well-known of today's Latin-American physicians. Dr. Wilson has contributed Chapter Fourteen: Ophthalmic Plastic and Reconstructive Surgery.

Richard W. Yee, M.D., is an ophthalmologist with fellowship experience in corneal and external disease. He is Clinical Associate Professor, Department of Ophthalmology at the University of Texas Hermann Eye Center in Houston. Dr. Yee has over 10 years' experience as an eye surgeon, specializing in surgery of corneal diseases with emphasis in anterior segment surgery, corneal transplant surgery, cataract and lens implantation surgery and refractive surgery. Dr. Yee is actively involved in Physiology Education and has authored dozens of publications in medical journals on the cornea, external diseases and refractive surgery. Dr. Yee was recently given an honor award by The American Academy of Ophthalmology and has contributed Chapter Eleven: Corneal and External Diseases.

Debra J. Yee received her bachelor's degree in Science in Marketing from University of Texas in San Antonio. She is consultant to Dr. Richard Yee on patient education, care and practice management.

Chapter One

The Evolution of Eye Care

Lawrence Lynn

Eye care evolved slowly over many years; then in the mid-twentieth century progress accelerated at an astounding rate. This chapter will offer the essential highlights of the historical development of the science of eye care. For those who wish more detail, we have provided a brief bibliography of resources in the Appendix.

Ancient and Classical Period

We begin with the ancient Near East, at the dawn of literacy over 6,000 years ago. We have very incomplete records of eye care. We know that medicine was a matter for priests, no doubt due to the amount of prayer necessary for patient healing, or for patient survival of the treatment. In the Sumerian and Babylonian empires a few maladies were known such as trachoma (a potentially blinding infection), night blindness, corneal ulcers and scars, and tearsac infections. A bronze lancet seems to have been used in the simple procedures.

Surgeons were highly regarded and well-paid. The surgeon received two silver shekels for treating a prisoner or five shekels for operating on a freeman, good wages indeed. However, while no such thing as malpractice insurance existed, an extreme substitute existed to discourage carelessness. The penalty for a botched operation on a slave was for the surgeon to lose his entire fee, bad enough; but if an operation on a freeman failed, the law called for both the surgeon's hands to be cut off, thereby preventing any further damage to anyone. No doubt this was the period during which Western Civilization first recorded the general principles of law which would wind up in the Old Testament, such as "an eye for an eye."

In ancient Egypt, the field of eye surgery was also a priestly matter. Egyptian culture produced no specialized surgical instruments and only a few writings on the subject. The oculist, however, was much honored, judging from a papyrus found in a pyramid at Gizeh in 1920. The writer also mentioned that a disease similar to pinkeye was prevalent and causing misery to early Egyptians. The only "surgery" performed was the removal of eyelashes scratching the eye, and tweezers possibly for this purpose have been discovered. Medications included copper derivatives, urine, saliva, honey, white of eggs, and the milk of a woman who had borne only boys. As elsewhere, the separation of science and magic was nearly impossible at the time.

About 4,500 years ago, Indian society had the most advanced ophthalmic knowledge of the ancient world. The early doctors recognized about seventy-five different eye problems. The penalty for poor surgery was loss of the surgeon's nose. Such refinements of treatment such as anesthesiology were completely unknown.

Even a type of cataract surgery called "couching" was developed (Fig. 1–1). The procedure involved first cleansing the body thoroughly for a day or two, using purgatives. After this, and following suitable entreaties for divine aid, the patient lay down and was told to focus on the end of his nose. Then a lightening-fast puncture was made with a thin reed, pushed through the pupil of the eye. The idea was for the reed to instantly push the cataractous lens cleanly into the vitreous cavity. Of course this crude procedure could also move the lens to positions where it could cause serious complications or blindness, but no alternatives existed. Miraculously, there were instances in which the patient actually recovered from this procedure with improved eyesight—and the surgeon kept his nose.

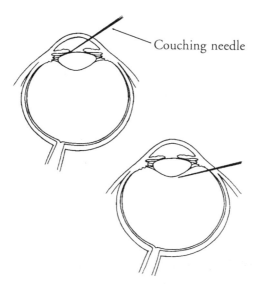

Figure 1–1   "Couching," a primitive technique to dislocate a cataractous lens, showing frontal and rear approach with a couching needle.

Eye care is mentioned in the Old Testament. The prophet Samuel felt that the religious rule of keeping the Sabbath holy and free of work should allow the key exception of emergency medical treatment for eyes. Frequently mentioned is the "evil eye" in the Hebrew writings and folklore, and in the holy Talmudic writings of its rabbis. Reference is made in the Talmud to the "majlis," the fluid believed to flow from the brain through the optical opening to and from the tear ducts. Preparation of salves was exotic. For example, the treatment of glaucoma was to grind a pre-dried scorpion, convert it from a powder into a paste, and apply this to the eyes. No records of success or failure from such efforts have come down to us, not surprisingly.

The most notable ancient Greek physicians were Hippocrates, Democritus, Celsus, and Galen. Their suggested treatments for eye maladies were fanciful in many cases. Notably here, myopia (nearsightedness) and hyperopia (farsightedness) could be corrected, they hoped, through jogging and the imbibing of recommended wines.

For middle-aged patients, these prescriptions no doubt added ankle degeneration and gout to their overall medical discomfort. One of the books left to us by Hippocrates is filled with information about eye care, much of it highly erroneous due to his lack of adequate anatomical knowledge. Democritus described the ciliary bodies, the iris, choroid, and pupil correctly in general terms, but in little detail. Celsus wrote that the foremost chamber of the eye included the lens and the iris, the *locus vacuus* (empty place). Celsus is better known for trying to clear out the many barber-surgeons who performed surgery along with haircuts.

Galen is famous for having named many of the presently used descriptive eye terms, such as the sclera, the retina, the aqueous humor, and the vitreous (see Chapter Two). He named them although he did not properly understand their functions. Galen discovered that the path of vision in the eyes ran from the optic nerve to the optic chiasm. However, he taught that the eyes contained materials called "hypochyma" which were carried along in the aqueous humor from the brain to the front of the eye.

In Rome, curved glass lenses to correct visual deficiencies were used for myopia and hyperopia. A wealthy Roman might carry a lens around with him in the way Prussian officers carried their monocles 1500 years later. The emperor Nero was said to use a precious stone as a lens to help him read. Paired lenses, as framed spectacles, were unknown.

The Middle Ages

For a thousand years or so following the classical era, there was almost no progress in eye care. Mythology continued to do well, however. For example, in Byzantine times the recommended treatment for the loss of aqueous humor in the anterior chamber of the eye following surgery was to bathe and partake of the vine, a clear carry-over from former Greek approaches to myopia and hyperopia. There were still no solid ideas about the anatomy and interrelationships of the different parts of the eye.

One might have expected that during the flowering of Islamic learning after 700 A.D., eye care would have undergone significant

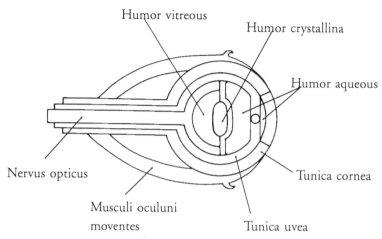

Figure 1–2 The eye according to a drawing by Alhazen, an Islamic physician.

advances, but this was not the case. However, and for this we are thankful, scholars preserved the earlier teachings of the Greeks by translating them into Arabic. An Arab eye surgeon had to receive a diploma in order to practice, a major advance. He was under surveillance by an inspector general. The Arabs eliminated the barber-surgeon altogether in the lands under their control, something not duplicated in Europe until much later.

A rough cross-section drawing of the eye has come down to us from Alhazen, a famous Arab surgeon (Fig. 1–2), which showed the lens, the optic nerve, and the cornea.

Alhazen's sketch is especially remarkable since few anatomical drawings of the eye or of other parts of the body were made by any Muslim physicians, perhaps because Islam unhelpfully prohibits the making of "graven images." A lack of such models was key to the limited progress made during the Islamic golden period.

Ophthalmology in contemporary Europe was just as primitive during the Middle Ages. A few medical schools were established in Reims, Bologna, and Chartres, but they used texts from the Arab lands which were essentially the old Greek tomes. Eye care held much lower prestige in Europe than in the Arab countries, and the field long continued to be dominated by the barber-surgeons.

Andreas Vesalius, a professor at Padua in Italy toward the end of the medieval period, incorrectly thought the lens was at the center of the eye, but he did know it was biconvex (Fig. 1–3).

He also understood that the iris pigmentation gives the eye its color, and knew something of the nature of the liquid aqueous humor. He was dimly aware that the retina was involved in some sort of photoreception process, although he did not understand the mechanism involved.

A major advance in eye care came about through the research of Roger Bacon, an Englishman who lived in the thirteenth century. After learning about the use of lenses for correcting vision, he produced the first known spectacles for patients to wear. Glasses became widespread in Europe by the seventeenth and eighteenth centuries. The very first eyeglasses were made of precious stones such as beryllium or emerald. Lenses for the less affluent soon were made of glass, manufactured mainly in countries such as England and Italy which had excellent glass industries. Glasses quickly attained an association with literacy, even scholarship. The famous portrait of Pope Leo X by Raphael in 1492 shows him wearing eyeglasses with concave lenses in a metallic frame. Martin Luther is said to have owned eight pairs of eyeglasses.

The perfection of glasses required several centuries more time, and their use to correct astigmatism did not take place until Young discovered the condition in his own eyes in 1801. Scientists such as Benjamin Franklin in Philadelphia developed the first bifocals so that reading or distant vision was possible without switching spectacles. The late 18th century may be considered the start of the early modern period of eye care.

Early Modern Period

Ophthalmology as a discrete branch of medical science can be traced to the time of Napoleon Bonaparte's Egyptian campaign in the last years of the eighteenth century.

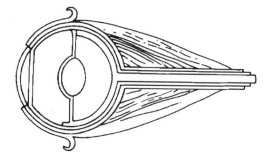

Figure 1–3 The eye according to Vesalius, a professor from the late Middle Ages.

Egypt, and indeed all of Africa, suffered from mass diseases and illnesses. Egypt was particularly well-known as a problem area. The lowlands in the delta and along the Nile were periodically flooded and created a perfect environment for malaria and other insect-transmitted diseases to develop and spread. It was also a reservoir of venereal diseases, as Napoleon's soldiers unhappily discovered. Among the worst afflictions were the terrible eye maladies collectively known as "Egyptian ophthalmia," of which two general types were described. *Ramad khafifi* was an inflammatory disease which was without complications; *ramad sadadi* was quite serious and generally led to blindness. The causes of these diseases were not known at the time. They were so pervasive among the general population that Egypt was called the "Land of the Blind."

When the French landed, initially no real attention was paid to the ophthalmias. It was thought that soldiers who suffered from ophthalmia would be cured by the passage of time or through elementary sanitation. This did not occur because the men had no resistance to ophthalmias. Within a few months, between one-half and two-thirds of all the French troops became afflicted with these diseases, some 20,000 of the 32,000 French troops in the field. *Ramad sadadi* produced severe inflammation of the conjunctiva, massive swelling of the eye lids, great pain, and a discharge similar to that of gonorrhea. Not until much work in the field of bacteriology and ophthalmology would it be discovered that these diseases were caused by a combination of *Hemophilus aegyptius, N. gonorrhea,*

Chlamydia trachomatous, and adenoviruses. For the moment, eye disease was a major component in the total catastrophe of the Egyptian campaign, and in Napoleon's abandonment of it as hopeless to rebuild.

Needless to say, the onslaught on the eyes of the French troops caused an immediate surge of European interest in ophthalmology. It became a separate field of medical science in France and England as well as in other lands. Curiosity, however, did not mean new cures. Old myths survived because there was nothing better available, and knowledge of the eye's anatomy was still primitive. Treatment continued to be based upon those used during the classical periods of Greece and Rome.

At the start of the nineteenth century, treatments of eye disease consisted of leeching, sweating, and purgatives, or counter-irritants such as poisoning with mercury. To prevent infection after surgery, especially after cataract extraction, bleeding was almost universal. Many patients went blind because of its weakening effect on the body.

Austria developed into the world center of all medical knowledge during the nineteenth century, including the theory and practice of ophthalmology. Johann Adam Schmidt and Joseph Beer were founders of this "Vienna School" to which outstanding students from England, Canada, the United States, Germany, and other countries came for training. Vienna's primacy continued until the 1920's, by which time other countries had developed their own centers for education and updating surgical methods.

Beer published important works on cataract extraction and corneal diseases, in monographs which were up to date on anatomy. He was the first to make the distinction between conjunctivitis due to gonorrhea, and iritis due to syphilis. These conditions had previously been considered one disease. He performed fragmentation removal of cataracts among children as opposed to simple extraction. Johann Friedrich Difenbach was the first to popularize the surgical correction of misalignment of the eyes. Traugott Wilhelm Gustav Benedict discovered the connection between eye disorders and diabetes. He was the first to teach the use of medications for dilation of the pupil, a major step forward. Edward Jaeger in 1855 discovered diabetic retinopathy, a severe retinal disease, and was partially successful in correcting it by treating diabetes.

In the very first part of the nineteenth century, English and French physicians generally refused to do ophthalmic surgery. Success rates were low, with associated threats to reputations from failed operations. Thus, here was a field much neglected through the choice of physicians themselves. Then matters began to change. James Wardrop popularized paracentesis, a surgical stab into the frontal cavity to prevent blindness through reducing extreme fluid pressure. G. J. Guthrie began to teach the use of silver nitrate in a salve to treat pinkeye. Across the Channel, Julius Sichel in France soon developed a surgical iridectomy technique for glaucoma. He also was the first to use ether systematically as an anesthetic for eye operations.

In the contemporary United States, Philadelphia, the largest city in the country until 1850, emerged as the center of American medical science. In addition to pioneering the manufacture of bifocal lenses, Benjamin Franklin had taught Americans the principles of optics and physics of light. The first optical shop was set up by John McAllister, who retailed whips and canes in addition to eyeglasses. David Agnew became famous for his theories about glaucoma and for his work on crossed eyes. William Edmonds Horner wrote landmark texts on optical anatomy, and taught the latest advances in his field to the ophthalmological students of his day. Henry Willard Williams became the first person to use a corneo-scleral suture to close a surgical wound after cataract extraction.

Cataract surgery could not advance until the anatomy of the lens had been completely learned. It was only in 1722 that physicians discovered that a cataract was just an opaque lens, and that it could be removed instead of couched. De la Faye designed the first knife specifically for cataract surgery. It took over 100 years for the "Daviel-St. Yves procedure" to become generally accepted, since antiseptic measures were not used until 1870 and local anesthesia for cataract surgery not until 1884. Residual cataract wounds were large and slow to heal.

The term "keratoplasty" was first used by Resinger in 1824 and defined as the remolding or reshaping of the cornea "to improve visual acuity." The first significant triumph in keratoplasty was achieved in New York by Kissam in 1838 when he used the cornea of a six-month-old pig to correct the eye of a patient with a defect called a staphyloma. The animal cornea significantly improved the vision of the patient at first but in time the donor cornea was absorbed into the eye of the patient, ending its benefit. Diffenbach later taught that the graft of any animal donor would be of little use for a human patient, and by the 1880s and 90s Amilian Adamuck and Ernst Fuchs and others concluded that only a human donor could provide material of any lasting value.

Modern Period

By the start of the twentieth century, the eye's anatomy was well enough understood to try out new ideas about ophthalmic surgery. The field of bacteriology had also advanced, along with the metallurgy to devise very delicate surgical tools and instrumentation. At last, the practicing eye doctor had the tools with which he needed to work.

For communication with the public, ophthalmology also directly incorporated verbiage from ancient texts rather than the use of more accessible terms. The merits of such new procedures as "corneal refractive surgery," including the procedures known as "refractive keratoplasty," were opaque to most persons outside the field when they were developed. For that matter, they still are, although the increasingly wide use of the new techniques is changing this situation.

The field of corneal surgery had been disregarded for the most part until 1937, when Vladimir Petrovich Filatov extracted corneas from human cadavers for insertion in living eyes with reasonable success. In the Soviet Union during World War II, many Red Army soldiers had received injuries to their eyes from Nazi shrapnel. While studying and treating these patients, Svyatoslav Fyodorov discovered to his surprise that many of them experienced improvement of eyesight as a result of the cuts into the cornea. Those who had their eyesight improved had received incisions in a sort of radial pattern. This led Fyodorov to study a severely nearsighted young boy who also had his eyesight improved after the scars from an eye injury healed. Fyodorov realized that specific kinds of incisions created flattened corneas in such a way that myopia was reduced. The status of refractive surgery received a major advance as a result of the work of Tutomo Sato in Japan, published in 1950. He made corneal incisions to attempt to cure the unsightly forward bulging of the globe of the eye. Later, Sato used incisions on the inside of the cornea to cure nearsightedness, as the peripheral incisions flatten the cornea. But because Sato made his incisions on the inside of the cornea, many of his patients went blind; and yet in some of Sato's operated patients their myopia actually improved and stabilized. With an 80 percent failure rate, western medicine therefore spurned Sato's work as dangerous and refused to examine it closely.

Soviet scientists were not bound by such feelings. Sato's procedures had worked some of the time. Therefore, research might clarify matters and increase the probability of surgical success. A number of studies were begun, and led to the development of consistently successful modern radial keratotomy (RK) by Fyodorov. Essentially, RK means the tracing of tiny cuts like spokes in a wheel, with the "hub" being the pupil. It was found that all RK cases helped nearsightedness, and better than 84% of Fyodorov's patients with seriously myopic eyes had their vision corrected to 20/50 or better.

When these results were reported in the medical literature, it created a sensation among ophthalmologists. After the procedure had been used in the United States for three years, the National Institute of Health and the American Academy of Ophthalmology commissioned a systematic evaluation of RK. The Prospective Evaluation of Radial Keratotomy (PERK) is an ongoing study. Thus far it has shown that in virtually all cases myopia is reduced by the use of RK.

The successes of RK have encouraged an explosion of research efforts in which surgery has played an ever more important role. Astigmatic keratotomy, using a different set of incisions into the cornea to moderate astigmatism, is being developed by Luis Ruiz with good results. In Latin America, José Barraquer in the 1950's worked out the procedures for what are called *keratomileusis* and *keratophakia*. In keratophakia, Barraquer used a *cryolathe,* a machine for shaping matter at very low temperatures, with a *microkeratome,* a device like a carpenter's plane for incising human tissue into extremely thin slivers. Frozen donor corneal material was shaped into a small lens, a *lenticule.* This was shaped with the cryolathe to fit the patient's eye and restore vision. It was fitted after a *microkeratoplasty,* a surgical procedure designed to shave off a minute portion of the patient's cornea, which was then sutured back into place after being lathed. It has since been learned that a synthetic lenticule can be made, perhaps altogether eliminating the need for tissue obtained from a human donor.

Even more exotic surgery is now possible. In application of *keratomileusis,* a *lamella* or thin leaf of the patient's own cornea is removed from the front of the eye. It is frozen and ground to the right shape and size, then sewn onto the bed of the patient's remaining corneal material. This is a very demanding and unforgiving procedure, for no error with the cryolathe is allowable. It can be a helpful procedure, however, for treatment of severe myopia or other related problems.

"*Epikeratophakia*" treats both hyperopic and myopic eye conditions. It involves the use of donor corneal material instead of the patient's own cornea as a donor lens, shaped to specifications and sutured on top of the patient's cornea after removal of the outer corneal layer of the eye. This is much like patching a car tire after a blow-out.

And there is more. Other developed procedures involve the use of heat from thermal probes, lasers, or radio frequency to shrink and steepen the cornea. This may be useful in the treatment of hyperopia.

All of these techniques can be done in the office quickly and are essentially painless for the patient. They are now becoming more common in the United States and elsewhere, as ophthalmologists become trained to do them.

A great deal of cosmetic surgery for the eyes and the surrounding tissues is being performed today. It is far from superfluous because one's looks influence health through buffering self-image. Successful cosmetic surgery, for example, in the life of an elderly woman can benefit her entire outlook on life. A lady of 75 or 80 may be restored psychologically to the age and outlook of a 55- or 60-year-old person.

Consider some advances in cosmetic surgery. *Blepharoplasty* is the correction of the baggy tissue of both upper and lower eyelids. Advances here in the materials used for sutures has gained so much ground that the required sutures are now minute and easily available. In certain situations, the excess fat around the eyes is removed from inside the eyelids, producing no visible scars whatsoever.

The greatest advance in cataract surgery was learned accidentally, in the same way that RK was discovered. During World War II, German Luftwaffe Messerschmitts and R.A.F. Spitfires were shooting each other down over the English Channel. The transparent canopies enclosing the British pilots were made of polymethylmethacrylate (PMMA), a tough petrochemical polymer plastic which shattered when hit by bullets. Fragments frequently became lodged in pilots' eyes. At London's Moorfield Eye Hospital, surgeons there noted to their surprise that sometimes the fragments of PMMA actually improved the vision of the pilot and caused little if any inflammation if left alone in the eye rather than being surgically extracted. It turned out that PMMA had a refractive ability which was compatible (indeed completely tolerated) by the human eye. This would eventually give rise to the use of PMMA for synthetic eye lenses. It is very common now to use lens implants in human eyes from which cataractous lenses have been removed.

Perhaps the most dramatic of all recent advances in eye care has been the use of lasers. These high-intensity, small-diameter beams of light have many practical applications. It was discovered, for example, that the laser beam could be directed into the eye for treatment of the retina. The laser acts like a mini-welding torch, similar to spot-welding. Lasers are used to patch retinal tears and detachments. In glaucoma, the normal outflow of the aqueous humor can be "enhanced" by a laser, much like a plumber "snakes" open a kitchen drain. Laser glaucoma surgeries can be done in the ophthalmologist's own office, eliminating any need for a long stay in the hospital and sometimes even a trip to an out-patient surgical center.

Conclusion

Ophthalmology has probably made more significant advances in the past fifty years than in the previous five thousand years.

In the future, the excimer and other lasers will accomplish procedures perhaps yet unknown at this writing. New drugs such as antibiotics may be developed to better prevent and treat infections, or possibly new drugs to prevent cataract formation, or new drugs to restore retinal and optic nerve function!

Judging from the way ophthalmology has accelerated its pace, it is not unreasonable to expect continued rapid advances in ophthalmic care. Ophthalmic surgery may well be regarded as less traumatic than a typical visit to the dentist. It is not inconceivable that the next century could mark a complete end to the use of external lenses to correct eyesight imperfections, and that perfect eyesight in all people will become considered a birthright.

Wrap-Up

- The medicinal discipline of ophthalmology was rudimentary and primitive throughout most of early recorded history. Eyecare remained primitive until the Napoleonic era when, because of large numbers of ophthalmic infections in French troops stationed in Egypt, eye health care became a much more important field of study in such centers in Paris and Vienna.

- Despite this impetus, even the anatomy of the eye was not well known until late in the 19th and early 20th century. This void prevented major advances in ophthalmic surgery.

- Much of the major advances in modern eyecare, including ophthalmological surgery, were achieved only in the past two generations. The pace of development became extremely rapid after World War II commenced.

- Most advances in cataract surgery, treatment of glaucoma, the entire field of corneal refractive surgery, retinal laser surgery, and much of the reconstructive surgery techniques are less than 40 years old.

Chapter Two

Anatomy and Physiology of the Eye

Warren D. Cross and Lawrence Lynn

The more you know about ophthalmic anatomy and physiology, the easier it is to communicate with eye specialists and for them to communicate with you. Understanding how your eye functions, and what could go wrong, is essential to obtaining superior eye care.

Introduction to the Eyes

In ophthalmology, the term "anterior" means front and "posterior" means rear. "Superior" and "inferior" are used to signify upper and lower. The "anterior-posterior axis" is a fancy way to indicate the front-to-rear pole of the eyeball. This "geometric axis" is one standard base point used by eye doctors and technicians when characteristics of the eye are discussed. The "equator," the vertical plane of the eyeball around its largest diameter midway along the geometric axis, is another.

By using these terms, any sort of position or angular direction can be clearly described. By convention, as you look at the eye from the front, the starting point when discussing distance around the eye begins on the right-hand side of the eye. "Zero degrees" is set by convention at 3 o'clock, 90 degrees at 12 o'clock, and 180 degrees at 9 o'clock. Therefore, when your doctor says that your astigmatism is +1.50 at 90 degrees, you now know the axis is up and down.

General Description

Much of what we know about the eye has been learned in the last couple of centuries through careful research by scientists in Europe, Japan, and the United States. In many cases the names of different parts of the eye and the orbit honor the scientists who discovered or most eloquently first discussed them.

The eye is roughly spherical. The bony tissues of the face which surround it are referred to as the *orbit*. The eye rests in the front half of the orbit upon a muscular hammock surrounded by fat and connective tissue. Attached to it are a set of six muscles, the four recti and two oblique muscles (Fig. 2–1).

These muscles are activated by nerves, which, along with several key veins and arteries, enter the orbit behind the eye through an opening from the rear called the *optic foramen*. The *optic nerve*, an electrochemical conduit, connects the eyeball to the brain. The optic nerve branches into approximately 1.2 million nerve endings.

The average human eye is slightly less than one inch (22 to 24 mm) in diameter. It is comprised of two incomplete spheres of different sizes affixed to each other. The front sphere, the *cornea*, is like a clear window on the larger posterior sphere, the *sclera*. The cornea is the part of the eye through which refracted (bent) light enters the eye. It, along with the lens inside the eye, alters light signals so that they will register properly upon the retina on the back wall of the eye. Approximately one-sixth of the surface area of the eyeball is taken up by the transparent cornea. This partial hemisphere has a radius of curvature of about 7 to 8 mm. The larger hemisphere, the sclera, has a radius of curvature of approximately 13 mm.

The sclera is white and can be seen meeting the cornea at a junction called the *limbus*. If the eye is properly shaped, and the lens normal and young, the eye will be able to register a consistently clear

Anatomy and Physiology of the Eye

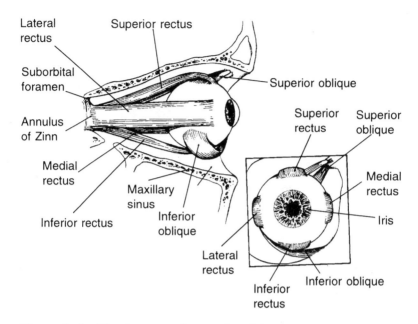

Figure 2–1 The six extraocular muscles of the eye.

image upon the retina for both far and near objects. But the power of the cornea, the lenses, and the length of the geometric axis can vary, yielding refractive problems or poor focusing of images on the retina. When images are distorted because the cornea and/or lens cannot clearly focus light signals perfectly upon the retina, the eye may be nearsighted: *myopic,* or able to see only nearby objects. On the other hand, it may be farsighted: *hyperopic,* or able to see well both at a distance and near as long as your lens is flexible and able to accommodate. Another possibility is that the eye will be *astigmatic,* in which the cornea is out-of-round and spoon-shaped, producing a blurred image because of two-dimensional warping. After the lens matures, if you are farsighted, you must use *plus lenses* to see well at distance and near.

There are three main compartments of the eye. The compartment closest to the outside front of the eye is called the *anterior chamber.* It is comprised of the cornea in the front and the iris or colored section on the inside. The place where these two parts meet

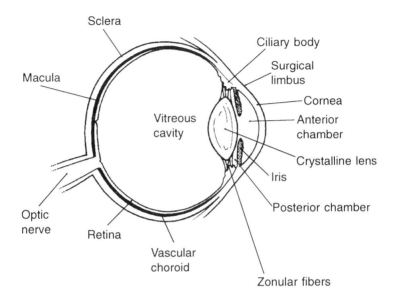

Figure 2–2   Cross-section of eye.

in the periphery is called the *angle*. A watery liquid, called aqueous humor, percolates through the eye providing nourishment and cleansing.

The cavity immediately behind the iris, in front of the lens, is called the *posterior chamber*. The third cavity, and the largest cavity, is the *cavity of the vitreous*. A gelatinous substance, called the *vitreous humor*, occupies this space and is attached to the retina (Fig. 2–2).

Cornea

The cornea is a truly amazing piece of living engineering. It is responsible for providing structural integrity and outward protection for one's eye, shielding it and the eye's complex miniature components from air, dust, cold, heat, light, and other external forces. It also helps to adjust the light which will be "seen" as it passes through the eye.

The cornea is responsible for about 60 percent of the initial refraction of light entering the eye. The lens refracts most of the remainder. The cornea is transparent, therefore *avascular,* meaning that it has no blood vessels. If it did, the tissue would be white and opaque like your cheek. The cornea is nourished by the liquid in the anterior chamber, the *aqueous,* and by the tear film on the outside. The cornea is where a contact lens is placed, should one be used to correct vision.

The cornea fits into the sclera much like a watch-glass fits into a wristwatch's bezel. It is tiny, only about 11.5 mm to 13 mm across. The border, or the *limbus,* is also covered by the beginning of the "skin of the eye," a transparent tissue called the *conjunctiva.* At its most central position, the cornea is 0.45 mm to 0.6 mm thick. At its margin it is slightly thicker. It is composed of five distinct types of cells which fuse together imperceptibly to form a transparent tissue. The entire epithelium is about five cell-layers thick, about one-tenth of a millimeter, and is the smoothest surface in the body. A smooth, healthy, clear *epithelium* is absolutely essential to clear, pain-free vision (Fig. 2–3).

The epithelium is the primary refractive "lens" surface of the eye. These cells provide a "waterproof barrier," helping to control how much water, salts, and chemicals pass into the *stroma* of the cornea, assisting to keep the cornea clear. The multiple layers of the cells, along with the tear enzymes, help protect the eye from bacterial infections. The presence of exquisitely sensitive nerves in the cornea assist in the eye's protection by informing you of pain, and causing tearing and blinking responses. The epithelial layer of the cornea heals quickly and, if abraded, is usually able to completely regenerate itself within one to three days.

Below the epithelial layer is "Bowman's anterior elastic membrane" which joins the epithelium to the underlying stroma. *Bowman's membrane,* unlike the epithelium, usually is unable to repair itself when damaged. However, it provides a substantial barrier to both infection and injury. Severe trauma or infections involving Bowman's membrane usually produce permanent haze and scarring. If damage happens to be centrally located, it may cause decreased visual capacity.

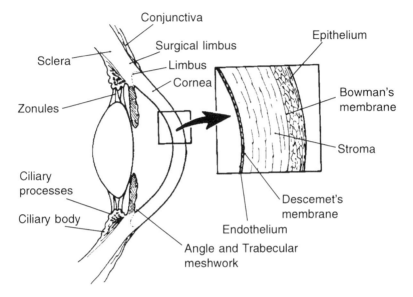

Figure 2–3   The corneal anatomy and its component layers.

The *stroma* is the main structural member of the cornea, representing 90 percent of the corneal thickness. It is made up of many perfectly organized, thin, transparent layers of a fibrous collagenous material, much like the matter of which the tendons in your hands, your fingernails, your hair, or a bird's feathers are made. The stroma helps give the eye its ability to refract images for the brain to develop into concepts. When all the thin layers work in concert, they give the eye most of its ability to refract the light signals transmitted to the retina.

The next inner material of the cornea is called *Descemet's membrane*. The Descemet's membrane is a very thin layer of transparent tissue of unique strength. It is also a good barrier to infection and chemicals and may be able to regenerate itself.

The innermost layer of the cornea is called the *endothelium*, a layer of cells with a vital function. They are minute pumps for the removal of water from inside the cornea. This pumping action to the inside, combined with evaporation from the front surface of the cornea, keeps the cornea "dehydrated" and "clear." If the cornea absorbed too much water it would become opaque and would not be crystal clear and would therefore be unable to transmit or refract light clearly onto the retina.

You are born with all the endothelial cells in the cornea that you will ever have. Since these cells do not reproduce and gradually degenerate during the aging process, they must be conserved and protected from accident, disease, and trauma. Any surgery done inside the eye is likely to cause loss of endothelial cells. If enough endothelial cells are lost, the cornea will ultimately become translucent instead of transparent. Sometimes this cannot be avoided. A routine cataract operation can cause a loss of five to 50 percent of the total number of endothelial cells. More than this could seriously jeopardize the future health of the cornea. Cataract surgery with severe complications can result in a much greater loss of endothelial cells. This is one of the major reasons why anterior segment intraocular surgery is so delicate an operation.

The corneal layers can be thought of as a clear windshield for the eye, and any damage may result in this layer becoming clouded, with reduced vision. One factor which can cause clouding is excessive pressure in the front chamber. Excess pressure in the eye, as from many forms of glaucoma, forces the endothelium to work under higher pressure than it was designed to withstand. Its cells will eventually break down and die; therefore, the pressure must be relieved or the cornea, as well as other parts of the eye, will cease to function properly.

Lids and Tears

The eye relies upon the simultaneous operation of several parts to keep the cornea functioning and in good health. Working hand in hand with the cornea to protect the eye from danger, foreign bodies, infection, injurious light, heat or cold are the eyelids of the eye. They are constantly in movement, blinking about 18 to 25 times per minute. Imagine the windshield wipers of a car. The driver must rely on the manufacturer's correct design of the window sprayer and wiper for the windshield to be of any help in foul weather or in a dusty road environment. When you are reading intensely or watch-

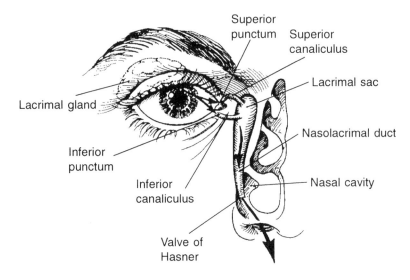

Figure 2–4 Diagram showing lacrimal gland and lacrimal duct system, which produces and removes the tears that irrigate and clean the eye.

ing a movie, your blinking rate decreases to about four to six times per minute. This is why if you have dry eyes, your eyes bother you much more when you read.

The tear, or *lacrimal*, glands located deep between the eyeball and the bony orbit at the upper outer corner under the upper eyelids pump tears into the eye to clean the surface of the cornea (Fig. 2–4). The tears have three major functions and are vitally essential to both the health and vision of the eye—so much so that "dry eyes" or tear infections and abnormalities represent 20 percent of most ophthalmic office treatments. The artificial-tears market does a business of more than $100 million per year.

Under normal conditions the ultra-thin tear film is comprised of three different layers from three different sources. The blinking eyelid applies this ultra-thin three-layer coat to both the corneal and conjunctival epithelial surfaces. One function of the tear film is to make the corneal surface optically smooth by "filling in" any minute surface irregularities. Second, by keeping the surface cells of the cornea and conjunctiva well-hydrated, tears prevent injury or death of the epithelial cell from dehydration. Last, the growth of microorganisms on the conjunctiva and cornea are inhibited due to the constant flushing and the antimicrobial action of the tear film. Concentrations of gamma globulins, antibodies to fight infection, are greater in tear film than in our blood. In addition, enzymes called *lysosomes,* which dissolve bacteria, are major defenses to keep our eyes sterile even though they are exposed continuously to a dirty world.

The tear film has an oily or lipid outer layer provided by the *meibomian glands* in the eyelids. If you pour a layer of oil onto water, evaporation of the water is greatly reduced. Our outer tear oil layer decreases tear evaporation in exactly the same way.

Lipids cover the middle water layer and are produced by the *lacrimal glands.* This water layer contains moderately high concentrations of water soluble salts and proteins. The deep mucinous layer of the tears, produced from the conjunctival goblet cells and lacrimal gland, attaches to the surface of the corneal epithelium and creates a smooth surface onto which the tear film can adhere. *Mucin* gives the tears their lubricating quality.

The side of each eyelid nearest the nose has a *punctum,* or duct opening. These four drains enable excess tears to be carried away from the corneal surface to the microscopic *canaliculi ducts* leading to the *nasolacrimal duct* inside the nose. This is why a person who is weeping needs a tissue to blow his nose.

In some people who have reached advanced age, especially when they also have an autoimmune disease such as rheumatoid arthritis, the production of tears is inadequate and the eyes can become very dry. The tear and salivary glands embryologically come from the same cells as your joint capsules, so when you have arthritis, you frequently have dry eyes and mouth. This is especially serious in dusty or cold environments where the eye, desperately needing tears to lubricate the cornea, can become painful. Fortunately, artificial tears can now be purchased over the counter for application several times per day or in ointment form for use at bedtime. While not as good as the real thing, since they lack the natural mucin or lipids of the body, they are helpful substitutes. Laser closure of the tear drain sites frequently helps many patients.

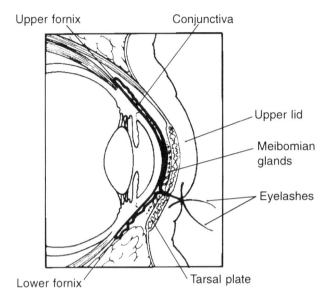

Figure 2–5 Cross section of anatomy of the conjunctiva and the eyelids.

Conjunctiva

The *conjunctiva* covers all of the inside of the eyelid and the outside of the eye, except for the cornea. Where the eyelid conjunctiva and the eyeball conjunctiva meet is referred to as the fornix (Fig. 2–5). The conjunctiva is a very thin membrane like the mucus membrane covering the inside of the mouth, lips and nose. Because it is continuous from the sclera curving around to line the eyelids, it eliminates the great concern of many patients about dislocating their contact lens and having it slip behind their eye to their brain. This kind of tissue is easily inflamed or infected, creating the condition known as *conjunctivitis* or *pinkeye*. These are irritating, but not especially dangerous conditions, if treated promptly, since they are superficial and usually respond readily to treatment.

Anatomy and Physiology of the Eye

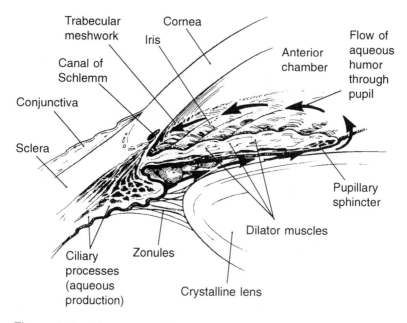

Figure 2-6 The anterior (front) chamber of the eye, showing the angle structure and aqueous flow.

Sclera

The scleral structure, the white part of the eye, is a tough protective coat consisting of highly compacted flat bands of collagen bundles which interweave in all directions and are interspersed with elastic fibers.

Anterior Chamber

There are three main compartments of the eye. The first and closest to the outside of the eye is called the front or *anterior chamber*. It is surrounded by the cornea in front and the iris and lens posteriorly. The bulk of the aqueous humor is contained in this space (Fig. 2-6).

Aqueous Humor

The *aqueous humor* is secreted by the back surface of the ciliary body at its base. It supplies water and nutrition to the corneal endothelium. The fluid is then reabsorbed in front of the iris at its base just behind the corneal-scleral junction in an area called the "trabecular meshwork." This largely aqueous material percolates constantly from its source in the rear chamber around the lens and through the black pupil, actually a hole in the iris, into the front chamber. The aqueous humor contains glucose, proteins and minerals, vital for nourishment of the lens and cornea.

Angle/Trabecular Meshwork

The *trabecular meshwork* is a tight-knit meshwork structure that filters the aqueous out of the anterior chamber of the eye. Damage or alteration of this structure, whether genetic, traumatic or due to inflammatory processes, results in the increased intraocular pressure termed "glaucoma."

Posterior Chamber

This middle chamber is the space behind the iris and in front of the vitreous humor. It contains the crystalline lens and is also filled with the aqueous humor.

Pupil

Contrary to common belief, the *pupil* is not an organ or structure. It is simply a hole in the center of the iris and is "black" because there is no light inside the eye.

Iris

The *iris* is in front of the lens allowing aqueous humor to percolate from behind it toward the anterior chamber. The iris contains the color bodies which give the eye its color of black, brown, green, or blue. Generally the lesser quantity of color bodies or pigment present, the greater the tendency for the eye to be green or blue. If there is a high level of pigmentation the eye will appear to have a brown or black iris. The iris contains two very important intrinsic muscles, the pupillary sphincter and the dilator. The *sphincter muscles* around the pupil edge controls closing the pupil, and the *dilator muscles* controls opening the pupil. The delicate balance between the sphincter and the dilator muscles, controlled by the brain, is what determines the amount of light allowed to enter the pupillary aperture. There is a constant equilibrium of pull and push between both muscles acting in concert with each other for the eye to be open enough to allow good vision but not too much to allow any damage. The iris opens and closes at the discretion of these two muscles and does so automatically to admit the right amount of light to furnish the image which the brain needs for vision. Many neurologic conditions such as diabetes, aneurysms and infections, as well as many drugs, legal and illegal, topical and systemic, influence dilation and pupillary response (see Chapter Fifteen).

Ciliary Body

The *ciliary body* is a very vascular body, consisting of the ciliary muscle and the ciliary processes. It is located at the base of the iris, and serves many functions.

The ciliary muscle anchors the thin collagen fibers called *zonules*, which are attached around the periphery to the outer layer of the natural lens of the eye. As the ciliary muscle contracts and constricts, these fibers relax or tighten the lens, thus changing its shape and the eye's focus.

The ciliary processes are tiny folds in the ciliary body, which are responsible for the production of the aqueous.

Vitreous Cavity

This is the third and largest chamber. The back of the lens is the vitreous cavity's front boundary; elsewhere it is surrounded by the retina, which lines the inside of the sclera. The cavity holds the vitreous humor.

The *vitreous humor* is a very thick, sticky, gel-like substance containing mucopolysaccharides, hyaluronate acids, and collagen microfibrils. In the young, normal eye this is a nearly solid gel which serves to support or hold the retina in place as a protective device against trauma and subsequent retinal tears and/or detachments. With advancing age the gel liquifies, forming pockets of water in a "swiss cheese-like" fashion. The collagen fibers tend not to be held apart and are therefore able to condense together. Eventually, if they become big enough and are in the visual axis, you can see them as grayish "floaters." The floaters may disappear after days, months, or several years. As the process continues, the floaters drop by gravity and are no longer visible because they are below your visual axis or line of vision.

Crystalline Lens

Light, after being refracted by the cornea, passes through the pupil and then onward through the lens (Fig. 2–7). The pupil, you recall, is just the empty space between the anterior and posterior chambers which functions like the f-stop on your camera.

The *crystalline lens* is one of the most unique portions of the human body. Its function is to further focus rays of light, which have been already partially refracted by the cornea, so that they reach the retina in such a fashion that it can interpret them. The lens is held in place by zonular fibers, which pull at the lens body by contractions of the ciliary processes. When the ciliary bodies pull the lens, it becomes more curved and the degree of refraction is increased, allowing us to focus on different distances at near. When the ciliary processes relax, the lens becomes flatter and refracts light received from a distance.

The ability of the lens to become more convex is called *accommodation* and is essential to bring near objects into clear focus. The inevitable loss of lens flexibility is called *presbyopia*. A common complaint of those experiencing presbyopia is that "my arms are too short" to read; it usually "strikes" at about the age of 40. The eye then may need an outside lens to make up for diminished natural capability. If you are already wearing one spectacle correction for

Anatomy and Physiology of the Eye

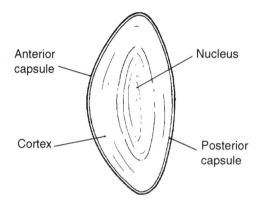

Figure 2-7 Components of the natural crystalline lens.

distance vision and you become presbyopic, you will now need bifocals—two lens corrections in one set of glasses so you can also see near objects well.

At infancy the lens is relatively soft and more liquid and elastic than when you are older. Because the eye is sealed and there is no way to remove old lens cells, with age the lens grows by adding layers. These are compressed into a tighter and more rigid nucleus surrounded by a cortex of fibrils not so tightly compressed. The nucleus will gradually lose its transparency with age and eventually become dark and translucent.

If it becomes sufficiently opaque, it will excessively block the passage of light to the retina. This is the process that evolves as a cataract changes from benign or insignificant into one which diminishes the quality of vision. A cataract can cause eyesight to vary and measure anywhere from 20/20 to an eyesight of 20/200 or worse, which in most American states is legal blindness.

An advanced cataract must be removed by surgery to restore vision, usually replacing it with a new lens or intraocular lens implant (IOL). Cataract surgery today is comparatively simple and painless, and can be done in 20 to 45 minutes. There is little left of the old post-operative therapies anymore, and recovery is quite swift (Chapter Five).

Retina

The *retina* lines the inside of the eyeball behind the colored iris, and is comprised of hundreds of millions of nerves distributed into nine layers, which also contain the vessels and photochemical receptors for vision. The retina contains two types of receptor cells which are referred to as the "rods" and the "cones." The largest number of receptors are the rods, which are estimated to be approximately 20 million per eye. The rods function best in low illumination, reaching maximum sensitivity after being in darkness for approximately 30 minutes. This dark adaptation or "shift" explains your inability to see when you first enter a dark movie theater, but also explains why you can see much better after a passage of time. The rods cannot distinguish color. They are black-and-white receptors, and are so sensitive that a person can see a lit match 14 miles away on a dark night.

Rods line the inside of the eye except for the central area which is referred to as the *macula*. The macula contains the cone retinal receptors which are responsible for color and detail vision. Cone cells work best in high illumination. The *macula* is located in the central retina directly behind the pupil. The tiny, central portion of the macula is referred to as the *fovea* and is responsible for our fine detail vision. Underneath the retina is the retinal pigment epithelium (RPE) layer which functions as a waterproof barrier, absorbing excess light and providing part of your retinal nutrition.

Once light signals have focused on the retina (Fig. 2–8), they are transmitted through the optic nerve located at the rear opening of the orbit through two sets of neuro-fibers. The "temporal neuro-fibers" are on the outside away from the nose; the "nasal neuro-fibers" are on the inside, toward the nose. The nasal neuro-fibers cross each other at a point behind the orbit called the *optic chiasm,* then extend to two relay stations in the brain called the *geniculate bodies.* From there, optic radiations extend to the *visual cortex* in the occipital lobe of the brain toward the rear of the head (Fig. 2–9).

The question of the nerves, veins, and arteries, which sustain the eye, is too complex a subject to go into here. Let us say only

Anatomy and Physiology of the Eye

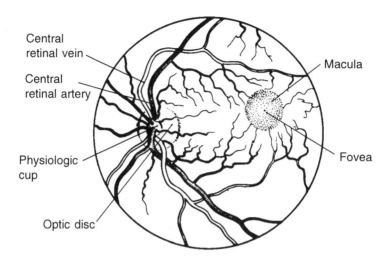

Figure 2–8 The retinal landmarks as viewed through camera or microscope.

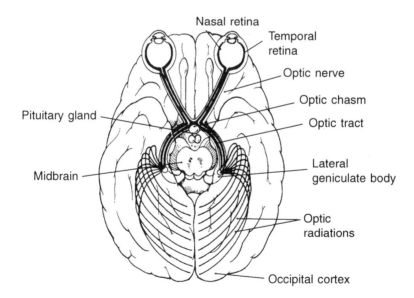

Figure 2–9 Connections from the eye to the true site of vision, the occipital lobe of the brain.

that the eye is served by a tremendous number of nerves, veins, and arteries which nourish every part.

Conclusion

Far from being the simple empty little globe it appears to be, the eye is an incredibly complicated device adapted to the careful manipulation of visual light so that it can be interpreted by the brain. All its parts must be in good working order, or else the function of the eye is impeded.

In visually oriented species such as man, a capacity to see well has always been of the greatest importance. A big contributor to man's evolution is the capacity of human beings to focus easily upon close objects, especially within arms' length, and the simultaneous availability of delicate, highly manipulative hands placed in such a position that their work can be closely supervised.

Wrap-Up

- The eyeball is about one inch in diameter.
- Eye movements are controlled by six separate muscles on each eye.
- The cornea is responsible for about 60 percent of our refractive ability.
- The corneal epithelium is about five cell layers thick, and is the smoothest, most perfect surface of the body. The corneal epithelium has a very high cell activity which allows it to heal rapidly, usually in one to three days.
- The retina has the highest metabolic activity/needs in the body. The heart is 50 to 60 times heavier than the eye, yet the eye uses one-third as much oxygen as our beating heart.
- The retinal nerve fibers, estimated to be 700,000 to 1.2 million per eye, represent 40 percent of the total fibers going to the brain. The nerves are compressed together so tightly (150,000 per square

millimeter) in the fovea that there is not even a capillary in the area for blood supply.

- Eyesight accounts for 90 to 95 percent of all our sensory perceptions.
- Corneal dehydration is maintained by water evaporation from the surface and the endothelial cells pumping water back into the eye on the inside.
- It is estimated that you have blinked 245,537,413 times by the time you reach 50 years of age!
- It is impossible to sneeze and keep your eyes open without blinking.
- There are 100 to 150 eyelashes in your upper eyelid, which is two times as many as in your lower eyelid.
- The crystalline lens becomes larger in diameter and thicker each year in your early years. It lives in an aqueous humor "bath" and does not have any blood supply.

Chapter Three

The Comprehensive Eye Examination

Stacey L. Brown, Warren D. Cross, and Lawrence Lynn

A comprehensive eye examination is necessary to determine the health of your eyes. The exam takes approximately one to two hours and is painless. This chapter is designed to "walk you through" a complete eye examination. We will explain certain tests, why they are necessary, and the general order in which they occur. A complete eye examination consists of your medical and eye history, several preliminary diagnostic testing procedures, and specialized testing, if necessary.

An old saying has truth: "The eyes are the windows to the soul." The eyes can also provide an immediate means of determining numerous kinds of medical problems. Since the eye is so closely interrelated with the body's general health, over 250 diseases and conditions can be diagnosed by examining the eye.

In the larger and busier offices, the preliminary eye testing may be performed by an ophthalmic assistant. An ophthalmic assistant is a professional with extensive training who performs many of the eye tests and who assists in evaluating the gathered results. However, the assistant is not licensed to prescribe glasses or contact lenses; or to make a medical diagnosis or perform ophthalmic surgery.

Chief Complaint (Why Did You Want Your Eyes Examined?)

The chief complaint is most likely why you came to the eye doctor. This complaint may not be easy to explain to the technician, but it is best to mention any and all eye problems or concerns. Maybe your vision is blurry, or your eye is hurting or itching. Maybe you want to be checked for glaucoma because your grandmother has glaucoma.

Possibly you have been having headaches, which are a "headache" for the doctor, because they have roots in so many causes. Cancer, misaligned teeth, injuries, and infections of the eyes, sinuses or brain can cause a headache. They can be related to eyestrain, excessive work in a bright environment, or repetitive movement of the eyes rapidly back and forth, such as in reading. Poor lighting, which incidentally does not actually harm your eyes, can also cause a headache.

Conversely, maybe you have no eye problems and want your glasses or contact lenses checked to see if they are still the correct prescription. Even if your eyes are perfectly healthy, it is best to have them examined every one to two years.

Medical and Eye History

You will then be asked about your medical and eye history. It all may seem like a lot of bother, and it does take time to compile, but when eyesight may be at stake, the broadest data base possible is essential. You are born with only two eyes, after all, and you must protect them as fully as you can.

Your medical and eye history should include when your last physical and eye examinations were and what was found, present and past illnesses or problems with your general health and eyes, and your surgical history.

You will be asked if you wear eyeglasses or contact lenses or if you ever have in the past.

It is also pertinent to know any health and eye disorders family members may have had, for genetic inheritance is an important part of expected health.

Medications and Allergies

The technician will need to document all medications which are presently being taken. This is necessary to ensure that medications are not causing an eye problem, and that incompatible medications are not prescribed by the eye doctor. Many medications can affect the eyes. Some can accelerate the formation of a cataract, some may aggravate glaucoma, and some may cause macular problems. Try to bring a list of your medications, including the frequency of use and the strength of each. It is also important for the doctor to be aware of your allergies to medicines, foods, or sensitivities to such medical accessories as surgical tape, iodine or lanolin.

Eye Muscle Examination

Several tests are performed to evaluate eye-muscle function. One of these is called the alternate cover test. You are asked to look straight ahead while the technician alternately covers each eye. As the technician performs this test, she checks for eye movement. The eyes should not shift back and forth or up and down during this test.

To further evaluate the eye muscles and whether the eyes work together, she will ask you to follow a small flashlight or penlight with your eyes as it is moved into various positions. This test is referred to as checking your "versions."

An imbalance of the eye muscles is referred to as *strabismus*. Strabismus is characteristic of "wandering eyes," "crossed eyes," or sometimes double vision, and is caused by a weak or overactive muscle(s).

Pupil Examination

This procedure involves a small flashlight or penlight, which is shined alternately into each eye to check whether the pupil constricts properly in response to the light entering the eye. If the pupil is unresponsive to the light, there may be a disorder of the optic nerve or retina which will require further evaluation.

Vision Examination

Your vision will be checked both at distance and at near. This examination will be performed with and without your eyeglasses.

If you wear contact lenses, your vision is usually checked while you are wearing your contacts. If your vision is less than perfect with your contact lenses, a refraction will be done while you are wearing them. This is referred to as an "over-refraction." This test may ascertain whether changing the power of your contact lenses will improve your vision (Chapter Thirteen).

To check your distance vision, you will be asked to read an eye chart which is 20 feet away. You will be asked to read the smallest line on the eye chart you are able to see while covering each eye independently. Your vision is then recorded based on the smallest line read. If your vision is perfect without glasses, which is referred to as "emmetropia," you can read down to the line on which the chart says 20. This is referred to as 20/20, which means that you can see at 20 feet what the normal eye is able to see at 20 feet. Degrees of lesser seeing ability, such as 20/80 or 20/200, mean that you can see at only 20 feet what a normal eye can see at 80 feet or 200 feet. Legally blind, in most instances, means that your best corrected vision in your "best eye" is 20/200 or worse.

If your vision is not perfect, you may be asked to read the smallest legible line on the chart through a device which covers one eye and allows the opposite eye to see through very small pinholes. This device is referred to as a *pinhole occluder*. If the pinhole effect improves your vision, you probably can be corrected to that improvement with corrective lenses. The pinholes correct for the refractive error of your eye by allowing only parallel focused rays of light into your eye. Your *refractive error* basically indicates the corrective lens prescription needed to best correct your vision. So remember, if you ever lose your eyeglasses or contacts, make tiny holes in a piece of paper or cardboard, and you can see as well or nearly as well through the holes as you would through your glasses or contact lenses.

The next step is to have your near vision checked by using a "near vision" card held at a comfortable reading distance (Fig. 3–1).

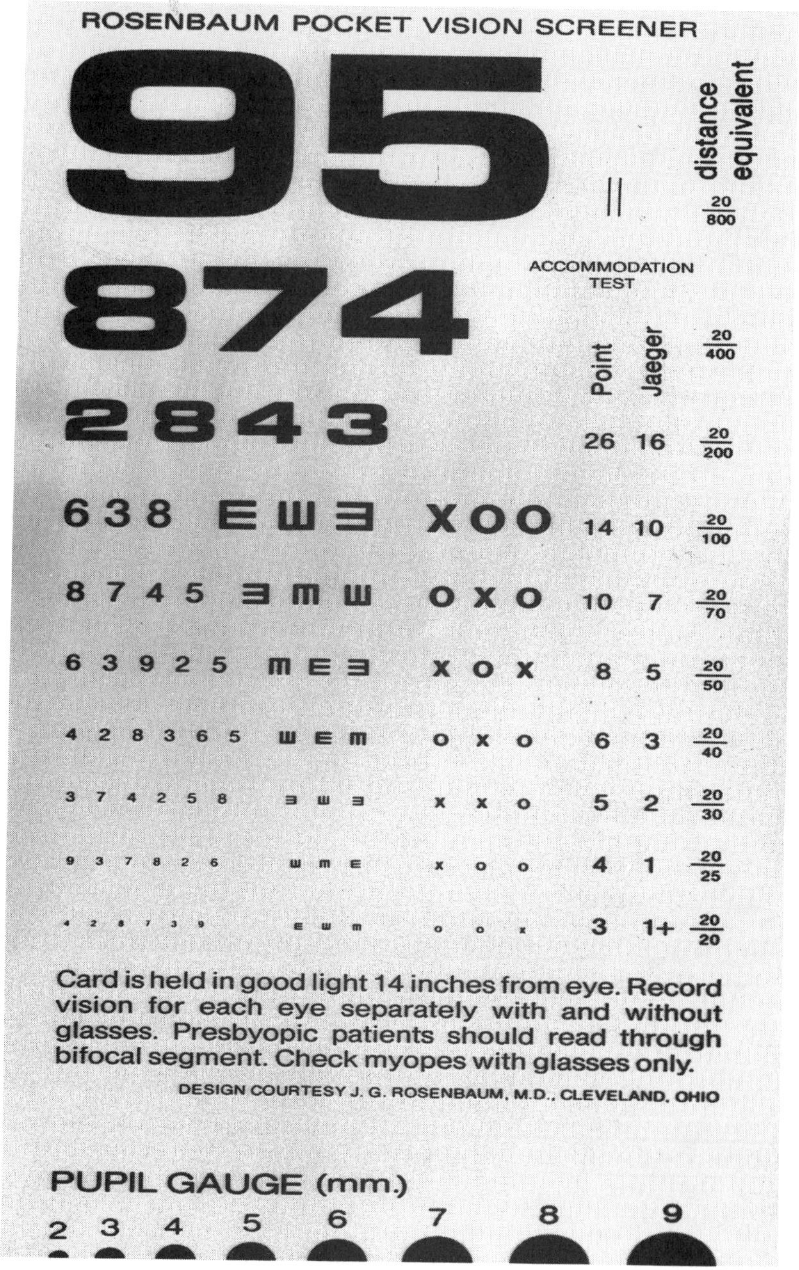

Figure 3–1 The near visual acuity chart. You may test yourself with and without glasses. Cover one eye while holding the chart about 14 inches away. Read the smallest line you can. Look to the right of the line you read and find your near visual acuity measurement.

The near vision card is used to check your near vision and is similar to a miniature hand-held eye chart, which contains phrases or lines of numbers in varying sizes. The procedure is the same as the 20/20 distance test, but necessary to ascertain whether reading glasses may be needed.

If you require corrective lenses for distance and corrective lenses for reading, you may be given *bifocals,* which eliminate the need for two pairs of glasses. You are corrected for distance in the upper portion of your bifocals, and you are corrected for reading in the lower portion of your bifocals. Some individuals require an "intermediate" area of vision which is not provided for in a bifocal. Intermediate vision is the area between distance and near, for example, the "fingertip" distance as you work at a computer or play the piano. Intermediate vision can be provided in a *trifocal* lens. A trifocal lens contains three areas of correction. You are usually corrected for distance vision in the upper portion of your trifocals, intermediate vision in the center portion of your trifocals, and a closer reading distance in the lower portion of your trifocals.

If you see less than 20/20 in any of these areas, your corrective lens prescription will then be determined. This procedure is referred to as *refractometry.*

Refractometry

If you wear glasses or contact lenses, their prescription will be checked with a lensmeter. Your present corrective lens prescription will be compared to the new corrective lens prescription. This comparison is necessary to ascertain whether a new prescription is significant enough to warrant a change in your corrective lenses. Of course, if there is a significant improvement in your vision with even the slightest change in your lenses, you will probably want a new pair of glasses or contact lenses. These decisions are based upon your visual needs—for example, driving, reading, and working.

If you do not wear glasses, and need them, you may be asked to look into a computerized automatic refractor. The automatic refractor is a quick method to determine your corrective lens prescription. The results given are then used as a guideline or "starting

The Comprehensive Eye Examination

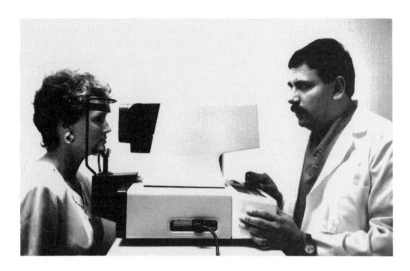

Figure 3–2 A Humphrey Automatic Keratometer for examining regularity or deviations in corneal curvature.

point" to determine your lens prescription. Another instrument used to find the "starting point" of your refractive error is the retinoscope. While you are sitting and looking straight ahead, the technician shines a light from inside the retinoscope into your eye. The movement of this light, referred to as a "reflex," is evaluated and various lenses are placed before your eye until the movement is "neutralized." Neutralization means that the corrective lens prescription has been reached. The retinoscope requires no response from the patient to determine the corrective lens prescription. It is often used in the evaluation of small children or individuals who, for whatever reason, are unable to communicate with the examiner during standard refractive techniques.

Next, as a guideline, to find your degree of astigmatism, your corneal curvature may be measured. This can be determined by a keratometer (Fig. 3–2). There are manual and automatic types available. While sitting, you are asked to fixate upon a light inside the instrument while the technician operates the machine. The keratometer can also be used as a guideline in evaluating corneal characteristics for the fitting of contact lenses, refractive surgery, and disorders of the cornea, such as keratoconus (Chapter Eight, Chapter Eleven, Chapter Thirteen).

Utilizing a phoropter or trial lens set, several lenses will be placed before each eye on a "trial and error" basis to determine which lens or lenses best correct your vision. The final outcome is written in prescription form and given to you for your optician or optometrist to fill, utilizing your old frames or new ones of your choice. If you prefer to be fitted with contact lenses, the prescription found during refractometry will need to be converted into a contact lens prescription. This conversion is also combined with other determinants, such as the type of contact lens desired, the shape of your eye, the relationship between your eye and eyelid, and your visual demands (Chapter Thirteen).

After your refraction, the internal and external health of your eyes will be examined by the eye doctor.

External and Front Chamber Eye Examination

Utilizing a slit lamp biomicroscope, commonly referred to as a "slit lamp", which is basically a microscope with special illuminators, the eyelids, tear system, cornea, sclera, conjunctiva, iris, and front chamber are examined (Fig. 3–3). This exam usually takes about five to 10 minutes or less, if no problems are found.

The slit lamp is used for close range examination of the eye, beginning with the eyelids, checking for growths or styes, flaking, possible infections, and adequately open tear ducts. The conjunctiva and the sclera are examined for signs of redness, irritation, infections, inflammations, foreign bodies, pterygiums, jaundice, injury and other problems. A frequently seen infection of the conjunctiva is called "conjunctivitis," more commonly known as "pinkeye."

The cornea should be crystal clear. It is examined for infection, inflammation, corneal ulcers, opacities, foreign bodies, dystrophies, "new" blood vessels and abrasions (Chapter Eleven). An eyedrop containing a yellowish-orange dye (fluorescein) is usually dropped onto the eye, for enhanced viewing with the slit lamp. When combined with the slit lamp's blue filter, any peculiar area is lit up brightly and is very easy to see.

The Comprehensive Eye Examination

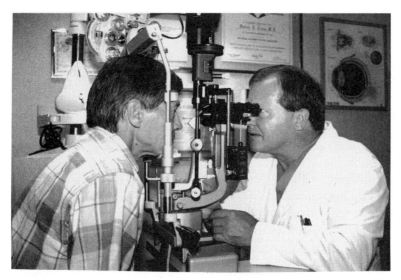

Figure 3–3 The Haag-Streit Slit-Lamp Bio-Microscope used for internal studies of the eye.

The doctor scans the front chamber of the eye for signs of inflammation, blood cells, and shallowness, which sometimes indicates narrow angle glaucoma. The examiner checks the iris for new or abnormal blood vessels, which may be growing into the iris. This condition is referred to as *rubeosis,* and may also cause glaucoma (Chapter Sixteen). These fragile blood vessels sometimes grow into the iris in response to diabetes and other vascular disorders.

Moving deeper into the eye, the lens is checked for signs of cataracts and flaking of the front surface of the lens. The back third of the vitreous chamber inside the pupil is checked for floating debris or "flare and cells," which could suggest a retinal problem. Benign conditions such as "gray floaters" or inflammatory material may also be found.

If all is well, your intraocular pressure will be tested next.

Intraocular Pressure Measurement

The intraocular pressure test is vital to appraise the present or impending existence of different forms of glaucoma. In glaucoma, there may be a decreased exit of fluid from the eye. The eye with glaucoma may be harder than normal, which raises the intraocular pressure. Pressure is determined with instruments called *tonometers.* This exam is a quick and absolutely painless procedure. There are several types of tonometers in use today, but the applanation tonometer is probably the most widely used. Prior to applanation tonometry, anesthetic and fluorescein eyedrops are dropped onto the eye. The anesthetic takes effect in less than one minute and wears off in about half an hour. The front surface of the anesthetized eye is lightly touched by a sensitive probe. The probe is calibrated to measure the softness or hardness of the eye.

Another type of tonometer is the "non-contact" tonometer, or "air puff" tonometer. No physical contact occurs between the eye and any part of the instrument. Therefore, anesthetic eyedrops are not needed. Instead, a stream or puff of air is blown against the cornea using an interval timer with infrared and photoelectronic cells to establish the point at which the cornea has been lightly flattened. It takes more time to flatten a hard cornea than a soft cornea and that is what is measured.

The results of tonometry are given in millimeters of mercury (mm Hg). A reading of 16 to 21 mm Hg is considered to be normal. Results of 21-30 mm Hg could indicate glaucoma. Measurements in excess of 30 mm Hg make glaucoma a strong probability.

The Dilated Examination

Usually after tonometry your eyes are dilated. If the angle inside your eye is extremely narrow or closed and/or your intraocular pressure is high, your eyes may not be dilated. This is because dilation, in certain types of glaucoma, can cause the pressure to immediately rise to a vision-threatening level.

Dilation is the beginning of the final phase of a routine eye examination and requires the use of eyedrops, which cause the iris to contract toward the periphery, enlarging the pupil. Dilation is necessary to examine the retina, macula, and optic nerve at the back of your eye, and to further evaluate the vitreous cavity and crystalline lens. The large pupillary opening gives the doctor a wide viewing area and enables him in most cases to thoroughly examine these areas. After dilating eyedrops, known as mydriatics, are dropped onto your eyes, they take effect in approximately 15 minutes.

Dilation will cause light sensitivity and may affect driving ability, which is why bringing along a "designated driver" to drive you home from the doctor's office is advised. After dilation has occurred, you will be asked to place your chin into the chinrest of the slit lamp. The doctor is then able to better evaluate the crystalline lens inside your eye to detect the presence of a cataract, and scan the vitreous cavity for floaters or debris that may not have been visible prior to dilation. This procedure takes only a few minutes.

The crystalline lens inside your eye should be crystal clear. If it becomes cloudy or opaque it is referred to as a *cataract.* Symptoms of a cataract may be decreased vision, poor contrast and color sensitivity, or excessive glare, such as seeing halos around lights and being temporarily "blinded" during night-time driving by oncoming headlights. Vision, when you have a cataract, has been compared to looking through foggy, dirty windows (Chapter Five).

The vitreous is a gelatinous substance that fills the back chamber of your eye providing firmness and support to the retina. With increased age, the vitreous sometimes liquifies and pulls away from the retina. This condition is called *syneresis* and can cause a vitreous detachment. A vitreous detachment is usually nothing but a nuisance causing you to see "gray floaters" that may look like flies or spider webs. But, since a vitreous detachment can cause a retinal detachment, a very serious condition, it is important that the retina and vitreous are examined promptly (by dilation) if you experience these symptoms. Symptoms to be wary of are multiple black floaters, flashes of light, or a "veil" or "curtain" coming across your field of vision.

The doctor will then examine your macula and optic nerve with a hand-held direct ophthalmoscope. The direct ophthalmoscope is a small instrument, which provides illumination and very high magnification for a detailed examination of the macula and optic nerve.

The macula is located approximately in the center of your retina and appears as a darker red area than the rest of your retina. The macula is responsible for your central and color vision. Damage to the macula, such as fluid accumulation, membranes, separations, or holes, can cause serious visual problems. If you cover one eye and put a finger directly in front of the uncovered eye, you can visualize how much a disorder of the macula can reduce your vision. You are left only with peripheral vision and will have difficulty seeing objects when looking at them straight ahead, if these objects are visible at all.

The optic nerve is the foremost "extension of your brain." It actually connects your eye to your brain, and transmits visual images from your eye to your brain. It penetrates through the back of the eyeball, which is embryologically a skin bag. The optic nerve opens up similarly to a flower and lines the inside back two-thirds of the eyeball, where it becomes a structure we call the retina. The optic nerve should be a salmon pink color with a shallow, central, whitish depression. This depression is referred to as the physiological "cup." Your doctor will record the size, shape and color of your optic nerve. Abnormalities of your optic nerve may suggest glaucoma, hypertension, vascular insufficiency (poor blood supply to the eye), optic nerve degeneration as in Multiple Sclerosis, inflammation of the optic nerve, increased intracranial pressure, sickle cell disease, and existence of tumors.

Next, the doctor will recline your chair so that you are lying flat on your back. He will then examine your eyes with an indirect ophthalmoscope. The indirect ophthalmoscope looks like a "coal miner's light" and provides a wide field for viewing the most peripheral areas of your retina.

A new technological development allows the doctor to use very small, high-powered, hand-held lenses combined with the slit lamp, in replacement of the indirect ophthalmoscope examination, to examine these areas of your eye.

When examining the peripheral retina, it is important to check for small hemorrhages, blood clotting, tiny holes (lattice degeneration), and diabetic changes (Chapter Nine).

Emerging and bifurcating from the optic disc are the retinal arteries and veins. The retinal arteries and veins are examined for any occlusions, straightening of the blood vessels associated with hypertension, or abnormal "new" blood vessels. An occlusion of a retinal artery or vein can cause a sudden loss of vision. This is referred to as a "branch retinal vein occlusion" or "central retinal artery occlusion." This is usually caused by high cholesterol, poor blood circulation, hypertension, arteriosclerosis, diabetes, and hardening of the arteries.

New blood vessels in the retina, which can become thin enough to bleed into the eye, may be caused from diabetes. This is referred to as *diabetic retinopathy*. Diabetic retinopathy can also cause serious visual loss and, if diagnosed or suspected, the eyes should be examined regularly.

The doctor's thorough inspection of the retina for detachments, holes, or breaks generally concludes the complete eye examination.

Conclusion

Unless further testing is required to make a diagnosis, the doctor has now completed your examination. Depending on the results, he is now able to give you a "clean bill of health" or discuss any findings and prognosis with you.

Special Diagnostic Testing Procedures

Special diagnostic testing procedures may be necessary should a problem with your eyes be found during the course of an eye examination. Should a disorder be found or suspected during a routine eye examination, the routine order of the examination may be altered in order to perform a certain test or series of tests.

Schirmer's Tear Test

Let's assume that you are a patient who wears contact lenses. You complain of the "dry eye" syndrome, or your eye's inability to tear. If so, your doctor may ask you to take a Schirmer's tear test. This test is conducted with filter paper strips which are permitted to remain in contact with the eye for five minutes after being inserted just inside the lower eyelid.

An anesthetic is used prior to this test in order to prevent "reflex tearing," which is the added tearing your eye produces when irritated. The Schirmer's test will indicate whether you produce an inadequate supply of tears, and if so, how little.

Gonioscopy Examination

If glaucoma is suspected or present, your doctor may want to examine your eyes with a goniolens. This deflects a beam of light into the various angles of the front chamber of your eye. The goniolens is used to study the angle structure or peripheral retinal areas of the eye, with high magnification. The entire angle structure is inaccessible in direct or indirect ophthalmoscopy examination. Your doctor wants to ensure the angle is anatomically open and not closed, as seen in a closed angle or narrow angle glaucoma.

Visual Field Examination

If glaucoma or a neurological problem is discovered, the examiner will check your visual field by confrontation. The examiner will sit in front of you holding a penlight and ask you when and from where the light source emanates. You may need a complete field test to locate blind spots and to determine your peripheral fields of vision.

Each of us has a "normal" blind spot about 10 to 20 degrees from the center of the field of vision. This exists because the retina over the optic nerve does not interpret light. This is not noticeable because the eyes overlap fields of vision and cover the gap.

The Goldmann Visual Field Test (Fig. 3–4) is a machine-assisted test to record when and where you notice light flashed into zones of the field of vision. The points at which the patient identifies the approaching targets are plotted on a chart and then manually connected by the technician to form isopters describing the unique capacities of your eyes to spot signals. An abnormal visual field may show a lack of potential vision in both eyes, as shown in Fig. 3–5. In many offices, computerized systems interact directly with you while testing your visual fields.

The Comprehensive Eye Examination 49

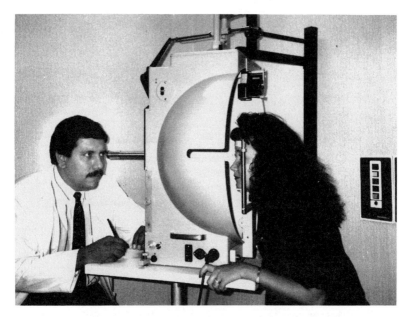

Figure 3–4   The Goldmann Visual Field Instrument used for measuring your peripheral vision.

Exophthalmometry Examination

If your eye protrudes abnormally, or if there is any suggestion of either thyroid disease or tumors of the orbit, the doctor will examine you with an exophthalmometer. This instrument is used to painlessly measure the forward protrusion of the eye.

Ocular Photography

If necessary, photographs may be taken of your eyes. There are several types. A *fluorescein angiography* is quite helpful in locating, diagnosing, and treating disorders of the retina. A fluorescein angiogram consists of injecting a yellowish-orange dye into the vein of your arm and taking a series of photographs as the dye enters and exits the eye, revealing staining and leakage of abnormal areas in the retina. The dye also produces a bright yellow color in urine for

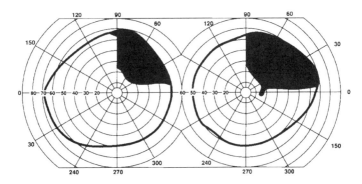

Figure 3–5 Goldmann Visual Field chart showing both eyes with a blind area of roughly one quarter of the visual field (upper right), a "quadrantanopsia."

about a day following the exam, and occasionally a temporary yellowing of the skin.

The doctor may also request photographs without the use of dye. These photographs are referred to as *fundus photographs* and track changes in the optic nerve in order to document glaucoma, tumors or lesions, and any suspicious areas in the retina or macula. *Slit lamp photographs,* with a special camera and accessories attached to a slit lamp, are used to photograph and document tiny, intricate problems of the cornea, iris, anterior chamber and the natural crystalline lens.

Photographs may also be taken of "droopy eyelids," lesions and tumors of the eyelids, and the muscle imbalances which produce "crossed eyes," "wall eyes," or "wandering eyes." These photographs are referred to as *external photographs* and are usually taken with a Polaroid or a regular 35 mm camera sometimes utilizing special zoom lenses.

Another type of photography, which may be necessary, is the *corneal endothelial cell count.* The corneal endothelium usually contains 3,000 to 3,500 cells per square millimeter in young eyes. As we age, these cells decrease in number at the rate of approximately one percent each year. If you have too few cells, your cornea may become painful, swollen, or hazy, and the world may look as if you were "swimming under water." An endothelial cell count is often requested if the corneal endothelium appears abnormal due to age, dystrophies, injuries, a thickened cornea, or if a particular surgery inside your eye is contemplated. This test is painless and is performed utilizing a high resolution camera with a small probe that lightly touches your anesthetized cornea (similar to tonometry). The probe is usually attached to a video camera and television screen, permitting you and the examiner to study and count your endothelial cells.

Contrast Sensitivity Examination

Special charts have been developed to measure the quality or parameter of vision which we call *contrast sensitivity*. These charts are useful guides if you have cataracts, optic neuritis, decreased choroidal profusion or blood supply, diabetes, and certain other retinopathies and compressive lesions (tumors, cysts, edema, etc.) of the optic nerve and/or the optic chiasm behind the eyes. The test is performed independently on each eye.

Amsler Grid Examination

If your doctor suspects problems with your macula or adjacent retina, an *Amsler grid test* is a simple and inexpensive test which may be performed. When focusing on the central area of the Amsler grid, abnormalities of the central retina are manifested by blurring, distortion or absence of the square. Many retinal patients follow their retinal progress at home by checking their Amsler grid daily (Fig. 3–6).

Night and Color Vision Examination

The retina contains two main retinal receptors, the "rods" and the "cones." The rods, located within the retina's margin are responsible for *night vision*. The cones, located within the macula, are responsible for *central vision* and *color vision*. Damage or loss of the rods results in diminished night vision. Damage or loss of the cones

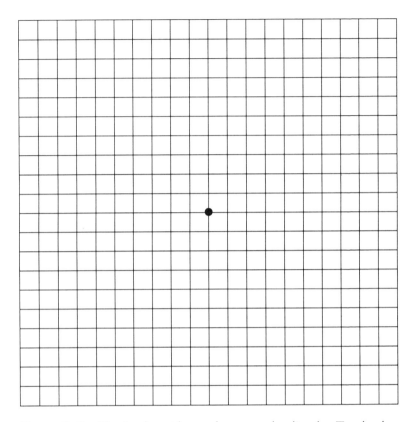

Figure 3–6   The Amsler grid to evaluate macular disorder. To take the Amsler grid test, cover one eye and hold the grid about 14 inches away. Fixate on the central dot. Is the central dot visible? Are any lines in the grid distorted or missing? Are the four corners visible? If any part of the grid is absent or missing, see your ophthalmologist for evaluation.

results in diminished central and color vision. The retinal receptors may be tested with the electroretinogram (ERG). The ERG measures retinal activity similar to the way the electrocardiogram (EKG) measures heart activity. Color vision may also be tested with the Farnsworth color disks, or the Ishihara Color Charts, which are a series of special color-dotted letters or objects within a group of colored dots.

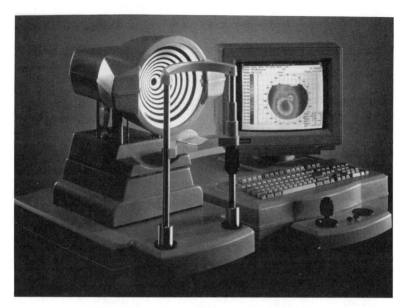

Figure 3–7 Computerized corneal topography instrument which measures every aspect of the cornea by projecting lighted rings onto the cornea, creating a computer analyzed map of the corneal surface onto the screen. (Photograph courtesy of EyeSys Laboratories).

Depth Perception Examination

Depth perception, essential in judging distances and exactly "where things are," may be evaluated if you have only one eye, a large difference in the vision of each eye, or a significant muscle imbalance. There are several tests available, the most commonly used tests being the fly test, the Wirt stereo test, the Worth four-dot test, and the biopter test.

Computerized Corneal Topography Examination

A sophisticated instrument, the *computerized corneal topographer* (CCT), is one of the newer diagnostic tools (Fig. 3–7). The CCT evaluates black-and-white rings projected onto the cornea, creating thousands of measurements to produce a surface map of the cornea revealing its power, curvature, and astigmatism. Computerized corneal topography is becoming progressively more useful in the evaluation of refractive and cataract surgical cases preoperatively and postoperatively. It is invaluable in diagnosing keratoconus (abnormal, irregular stretching of the cornea) and certain other corneal conditions. It is also an invaluable aid in fitting contact lenses and in follow up care after corneal transplantation and grafting.

Ultrasonography Examination

In opaque eyes (eyes you are unable to see out of and, consequently, eyes the doctor is unable to see into), the ultrasonography instrument uses sound waves of high frequency to penetrate tissues opaque to light to determine growths or retinal disorders undetectable by X-ray or ophthalmic examination. Two waves are typically used, an A-wave and a B-wave. An A-wave is a single beam linear impulse, which measures the length of the eyeball and indicates the position for the natural lens, which is necessary to calculate intraocular lens implant powers. A B-wave is a radiating wave used to detect tumors of the orbit, which cannot be identified by any other means, especially malignancies of the choroid, retinal detachments, hemorrhages, and foreign bodies. A CAT scan or an MRI (Magnetic Resonance Imaging) may also be used for this purpose.

Now you've experienced what a real comprehensive eye examination is like. See, it really is very interesting, informative and crucial to good health and vision!

Wrap-Up

- Approximately 250 diseases can be diagnosed by your ophthalmologist during a complete eye examination.
- If you are nearsighted, or have diabetes or glaucoma, you will need to have your eyes examined on a regular basis.

- If your eyes are "normal" and you see 20/20, you should have your eyes examined every two to three years after the age of 40, and approximately every year after the age of 60.
- The "chief complaint" or "chief visual complaint" is usually the reason why you came to have your eyes examined. Making a few notes regarding your condition prior to seeing your doctor is wise.
- For thorough documentation of your condition, it is important that you provide your eye doctor with your complete medical and eye history. This should include past or present conditions, treatments, and surgeries. It is also helpful to know your blood relatives' medical and eye history.
- It is important for your doctor to know the medications you take and the frequency and dosage of each. Again, a list may be necessary.
- You will also be asked if you have allergies to medications, foods, or medical accessories such as tape or gauze.
- Red/green color deficiencies are present in approximately 8 percent of all males and approximately one-half to one percent of all females.

Chapter Four

Refraction, Optics, and Eyeglasses

Warren D. Cross and Lawrence Lynn

If your cornea and lens are round and of the correct power, light will focus on a single point in your eye (Fig. 4–1). Errors in vision are often produced by the following: a slightly skewed eye curvature, erroneous focusing capacities of the cornea or lens, or an abnormally long eyeball. These errors are mostly due to heredity and age. Vision in these cases is optically correctable by glasses or contact lenses. Pathological refractive errors may require very thick glasses or contact lenses, which leave patients seeking surgical treatment.

Types of Refractive Errors

In *emmetropia,* or perfect eyesight, the focused image of an object falls precisely onto the retina. If the retinal image is not focused on the retina, vision will be blurred, resulting in a condition known as *ametropia.* In nearsightedness, or *myopia,* the length of the eyeball is longer than normal and/or the cornea is relatively steep, such that the retinal image falls in front of the retina. In farsightedness, *hyperopia,* the length of the eyeball is shorter than normal and/or the cornea is relatively flat and the retinal image falls behind the

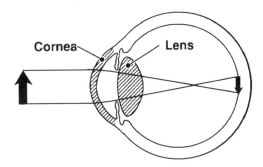

Figure 4–1   The eye's cornea and its natural crystalline lens together determine its refractive capability. Figure 4–1 shows the normal eye with the image focused on the retina.

retina. For myopia, since the image is in front of the retina, the image must be "pushed" back to the retina with a concave lens. In hyperopia, the image must be "pulled forward" to the retina with a convex lens. When the refractive power of the eye is different in different planes, the condition is called *astigmatism*. *Toric lenses* prescribed to treat astigmatism are cut to answer this exotic requirement.

When the power of the two eyes is different, the condition is called *anisometropia*. If the difference is significant, balanced correction requires contact lenses or refractive surgery.

The eye's natural lens can increase or decrease its focal power depending upon need, and depending upon the distance of the object from the eye. This alteration in the refractive power of the lens is accomplished by changing the curvature through the use of the ciliary muscles surrounding it. If there is an abnormality with this mechanism, or with a function known as *accommodation*, (Fig. 4–2A, Fig. 4–2B), you will have difficulty seeing either near or distant objects.

The ability of the eye to focus at different distances is controlled to some extent by the size of the pupil. The smaller the pupil's size, the greater the depth of field. Chromatic aberration, the scattering of light which causes fuzzy images, is also reduced by the pupil's smaller sizes. The smaller the pupil, the fewer optical prob-

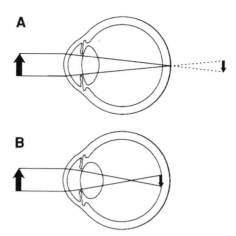

Figure 4–2 Accommodation of the lens.
(A) The image is focused behind the retina and vision is not clear.
(B) The lens accommodates (becomes more round) and focuses the image clearly onto the retina.

lems experienced. Although there are fewer optical problems with a smaller pupil, a smaller pupil will also decrease the amount of light entering your eye, which may cause difficulties with vision in dim illumination.

How We Focus Light

The term "vergence" is used to express the convergence or divergence of a cluster of rays while entering or leaving a lens. The unit used in measuring this is the *diopter,* or the reciprocal of the distance from the lens to the rays' focus, usually measured metrically. In other words:

$$\frac{\text{DIOPTERS OF POWER}}{} = \frac{1 \text{ METER}}{\text{FOCAL LENGTH IN METERS}}$$

For example, when you thread a needle, you hold it approximately 14 inches away (about one-third of a meter) from your face. You need three diopters of additional power either provided by

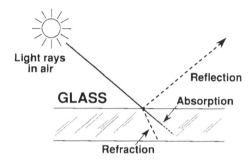

Figure 4–3 Light waves impinging upon a different medium will be partially reflected, partially refracted or bent, and partially absorbed by the new medium.

reading glasses ("readers") or by additional accommodation of your own lens to see clearly.

The total refractive power of the eye is approximately 60 diopters, of which roughly 40 is provided by the cornea and 20 by the lens. By calculation, your eye is about 24 mm long.

"Visible light" for human beings is the radiation within that set of electromagnetic wavelengths that the eye interprets. We cannot "see" longer wavelength infrared rays and shorter-wavelength ultraviolet rays and X-rays.

Electromagnetic radiation released from a source travels outward as rays, each ray on an individual diverging pathway. This diverging of the rays may not be readily evident if the radiation source is very large and close, or so far away that the rays finally reaching you have paths nearly parallel with one another. It is the distance from the point of origin which in part determines the amount of optical manipulation necessary to focus rays into a sharp image.

When rays of any wavelength travel from one medium into another, certain changes take place. The rays are partially absorbed, partially reflected, and partially *refracted,* or bent (Fig. 4–3). This last aspect is of great interest to the eye doctor, since refraction is the primary job of the eye.

The *refractive index* describes the amount that rays bend after passing through the interface of two media, such as from air into a

Refraction, Optics, and Eyeglasses

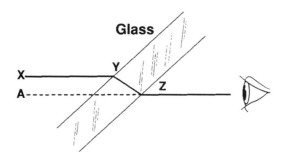

Figure 4–4   Refraction through a glass plate. Light ray XYZ is refracted at point Y, from air to glass, and at point Z, back to air. The actual light source, point X, appears to come from point A.

pane of glass or into water. This is why a fish in the water or a coin in the swimming pool is not where it appears to be when you attempt to spear the fish or dive into the pool to retrieve the coin. The medium with a higher refractive index is called the "denser" medium; the one with the lower refractive index is called the "rarer" medium (Fig. 4–4). When light starting from a rarer medium passes through a denser medium, the refracted ray is bent toward the "norm," or where an unrefracted ray would have been travelling from the source if uninfluenced by the denser medium. The "angle of incidence" at the surface of the denser medium is greater than the "angle of refraction" it passes through. As the ray exits into a medium with the original index of refraction, and if the interface surface is parallel to the original surface, as in a glass window pane, the ray is angled back onto its original course, but not in the same plane.

Let's consider this in a different way. Rarely in nature will one find media with exactly parallel front and back surfaces, such as in glass window pane. If the surfaces of a medium are not parallel to one another, any section of it can be thought of as a "prism." Consider a prism in its purest form, a triangle, and a ray passing through it after originating in a rarer medium (Fig. 4–5). Since the ray's initial angle of incidence on the prism is different from the angle of incidence as it exits, the ray does not return to its original

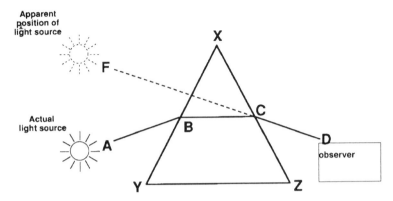

Figure 4–5 Refraction by prism XYZ where the apex is at point X. When light, point A, is refracted through the prism XYZ, the position of the actual light source, point A, will appear to the observer to be at point F.

course. This principle is used in making spectacles, which actually are prisms of graduated thicknesses which refract light toward the eye's pupil.

Each wavelength of electromagnetic radiation has its own characteristics and different degrees of refraction in various media. When radiation visible to the human eye travels through a prism, refraction splits it up into colors. This phenomenon is called "dispersion." Violet and blue light waves are the shortest and fastest, and the most readily bent; orange and red waves are longer and slower, and least readily bent. Diffraction is what produces a rainbow when sunlight passes through water droplets, for these act as small prisms and present us with the seven basic colors: violet, indigo, blue, green, yellow, orange, and red. Sometimes this set of colors is identified as the acronym formed from their first letters, or the *vibgyor*.

The rainbow effect also can be created within the eye. When the cornea is swollen from acute glaucoma, or in certain types of cataracts, there is an accumulation of water droplets inside the cornea or lens, and patients sometimes complain of seeing colored rings or halos around light sources.

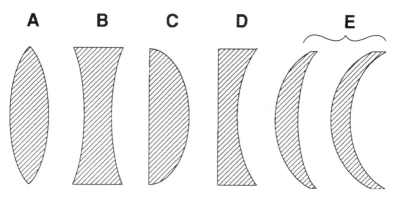

Figure 4–6 Various types of lenses.
(A) Biconvex lens.
(B) Biconcave lens.
(C) Plano-convex lens.
(D) Plano-concave lens.
(E) Meniscus lenses.

The eye doctor takes the matter of light sources into account when deciding refractions. Despite inventions which have permitted illumination of the night, human beings fundamentally are diurnal, daytime-living creatures for whom *sun*light is the normal electromagnetic environment the eye interprets. This is a "red" light source and daylight is ordinarily the eye doctor's baseline when prescriptions for lenses are made. A prescription can be adapted to other light sources—for example, the "blue" light of night—simply by varying the characteristics of the lens. Human vision being what it is, one might wonder why blue-light mercury vapor street lights are ever used, as compared with yellow sodium vapor street lights. The blue light is a shorter wavelength, which focuses quicker, tending to make us nearsighted at night. The answer lies in economics, not an interest in optimal vision.

A number of prism shapes have been devised to refract light for various purposes. Most lenses are round, or nearly so, but in cross-section they can be machined into biconvex, biconcave, plano-convex, plano-concave, or meniscus shapes (Fig. 4–6A-E). Circular

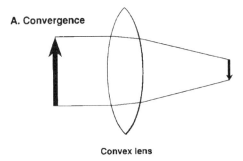

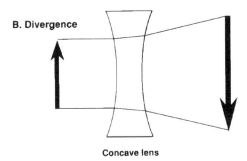

Figure 4–7   Convex and concave lenses.
(A) Convex or plus lenses converge the rays of light from a target (light source).
(B) Concave or minus lenses diverge the rays of light from a light source.

lenses have equal refractive powers in all quarters, aimed at a single spot. The classic example is the convex magnifying lens which "spreads" rays so that an image seems larger, or which can be used to focus rays intensely enough to produce a flame.

Convex surfaces bring light rays together to a point, and the lenses which produce this effect are called plus lenses (Fig. 4–7A). Concave surfaces cause rays to diverge, and the lenses which produce this effect are called minus lenses (Fig. 4–7B). The power of a lens is determined by the length of the radius of curvature, the steepness or flatness of its surfaces, and by the index of refraction.

A one-diopter lens will focus parallel light rays at a distance of one meter, a two-diopter lens will focus parallel light rays at a distance of one-half meter, and a four-diopter lens will focus parallel light rays at one-fourth of a meter, or about ten inches. If you are "six diopters nearsighted," you are twice as nearsighted as another person who is "three diopters nearsighted." You need a "minus" lens of twice the strength to correctly diverge and focus the rays of light entering your eye. The opposite is true for the farsighted patient, who instead needs a "plus" lens to add convergence power and help the eye to focus properly.

Partially cylindrical lenses are used to correct astigmatism in the eye. Imagine a solid cylindrical prism, then a single lengthwise slice taken from it. On the slice there is one curved surface and one plane surface. Cylindrical lenses have refractive power only in one meridian, that is, at right angles to the axis of the cylinder. If you shine a ray through this lens you will get a "line of focused light." Just as with circular lenses, cylindrical lenses can be convex (plus) or concave (minus).

When the image size created by a lens is larger than the object size, it is called *magnification;* when the image size is smaller than the object size, it is called *minification*. Magnification is created by convex (plus) circular surfaces. These may also be convex spheres or convex cylinders. Minification is created by concave (minus) lenses, which also may be spheres or cylinders.

Magnification or minification also vary according to the distance of the object and the image from the lens. Magnifying aids are used by patients with subnormal vision. These are called *low vision aids,* which may be telescopes for distance or various types of magnifiers for near vision.

Let us now consider basic vision problems and their correction.

Hyperopia (Farsightedness)

Approximately 15 percent of the world's population is naturally hyperopic, or farsighted. A *hyperopic eye* may be only a millimeter shorter than a normal eye, or may have a flatter cornea. Hyperopia is seen in 90 percent of children up to the age of five years, dropping to about 15 percent by age 16. After that, the eye retains normal status until age 50 or 60 and then the eyes begin to develop myopia or hardening in the nucleus or center of the lens.

Every millimeter of shortening of the eye results in two diopters of hyperopia. Six diopters of hyperopia is defined as the upper limit of simple, or acceptable hyperopia. In a young person this degree of hyperopia can be overcome simply by exercising or utilizing the ciliary muscle. Sometimes the effort is great enough to produce simultaneous convergence of the two eyes, a phenomenon called *accommodative convergence.* In children, if accommodative convergence is excessive, it can result in "cross-eyes." Some children are predisposed to cross-eyes due to heredity; in some societies cross-eyes are regarded as an attractive trait and worth cultivating. A person with *convergent strabismus* may require glasses, possibly with bifocals, for those societies who find it unattractive and an impairment to sight.

Some cases of hyperopia are caused when the corneal curvature is too flat to focus light onto the retina. Alternatively, the human lens may be abnormal or even removed as the result of cataract surgery. This condition is called *aphakia* and results in the most severe type of hyperopia. In the case of diabetes mellitus when there is fluctuation of the blood sugar level, the refractive index of the lens or vitreous can change and produce visual fluctuations.

These fluctuations may be your or your doctor's first clues about your diabetes. If hyperopia cannot be overcome through exercising the ciliary muscle, it is called *absolute hyperopia* and must be corrected with lenses (Fig. 4–8A-C) for a person to see well.

Myopia (Nearsightedness)

Nearsightedness refers to seeing clear objects at close range but being unable to see objects clearly at a distance (Fig. 4–9A–C). This can be caused by an abnormally steep corneal curvature and/or by excessive length of the eyeball. Myopia is an extremely common problem and affects up to 25 percent of the entire world's population.

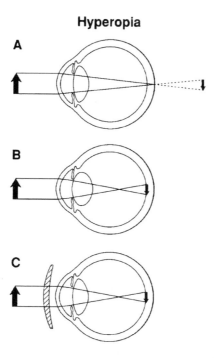

Figure 4–8   Hyperopia—farsightedness.
(A) The light rays from the target seen focused behind the retina.
(B) Accommodation has corrected the focus in a young person but can create a stress or headache.
(C) A spectacle lens corrects the focus.

Simple myopia often starts in the pre-teen years. During puberty, myopia increases rather rapidly as the face, skull and eyes grow in size, which results in frequent changes of lens prescriptions. At approximately the age of 20 the eye stabilizes. There appears to be some weak evidence that wearing contact lenses stops or minimizes the progress of myopia in children and young teenagers. Contacts have no influence on the progress of myopia in adults. But heavy reading, especially in poor lighting situations, appears to increase nearsightedness.

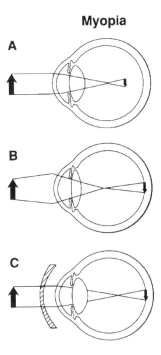

Figure 4–9　Myopia—nearsightedness.
(A) The image is focused in front of the retina from a far object.
(B) From a near object, the focus is perfect on the retina.
(C) A spectacle lens can focus the far rays (distance vision) to a proper focus on the retina.

If the myopia steadily continues to increase past age 20, it is defined as *progressive myopia* or, if excessive, *pathological myopia*. This condition may be associated with other ocular abnormalities and complications, like glaucoma, keratoconus, or retinal detachment. If you have progressive myopia, you should have a dilated eye examination at least once a year to make sure that your retina has not become detached or torn by the continual stretching of the eyeball as you mature. Occasionally, an ophthalmologist may need to treat these weak spots with laser or other procedures.

Unlike hyperopia, the intraocular muscles cannot change the internal focusing power of the lens to help overcome the problem. Myopia is now often treated with radial keratotomy or other refractive surgical procedures, which eliminate or decrease the need for either glasses or contact lenses.

In children, sometimes myopia may be associated with *divergent strabismus,* where the eyes are aimed too wide, the opposite of convergent strabismus in the case of hyperopia. This again can be corrected to some extent by glasses alone. If the divergent strabismus cannot be corrected completely with glasses, surgery on the eye muscles may be appropriate. In very unusual types of extremely high degrees of myopia, it can be corrected by surgical removal of the eye's lens. Since the eye with high myopia actually may also have degenerative retinal problems, this operation should not be taken lightly or as a first choice of treatment. It certainly is best performed in consultation with a retinal specialist.

Astigmatism

The third most important refractive problem is *astigmatism,* in which there is no single point of focus of the retinal image. The condition is produced by the refractive power of the cornea not being spherical or not of the same "roundness" in all meridians. The cornea, rather than being spherical like a basketball, has two different radii of curvature, like a football. Like myopia and hyperopia, astigmatism can result from an abnormal and irregular refractive index of the internal natural lens, as in cases of cataract formation or from the tilting of the lens inside the eye. Astigmatism is corrected by cylindrical lenses referred to as toric lenses.

Glasses Considerations

When a vision problem is in the process of correction, it is essential to communicate to your doctor exactly what you feel you need. Reading (or bifocal) lenses can enable you to read at only one particular range. If you and your doctor do not choose that particular range correctly, you won't be able to read, sew, write, or play the piano to your satisfaction.

You can pick up over-the-counter reading glasses at the drug store to see which is the best for you. These readers work best if both eyes are of equal refractions with no significant astigmatism in either eye. Choose the lowest power with which you can manage. You can certainly see better with higher power lenses, but stronger lenses may soon produce discomfort or headaches and require you to hold objects or to read at much closer distances than you wish.

Until plastics became available, eyeglasses were literally and exclusively made out of glass. Glass lenses were prone to shattering, and the stronger lenses tended to be rather heavy. While glass is still used, plastics are the material of choice for most patients.

Plastic lenses are very light but scratch easily unless protected by a scratch-resistant coating. For sport and for use by children, polycarbonate lenses are appropriate because they are especially resistant to breaking. A problem with these lenses, compared with regular plastic lenses, is color alteration.

You can have a lens made that has different powers within different areas. Limitation of the visual field with spectacle lenses may be produced by frame size or assigning the refractive power of the lens to a small portion of it. An instance of this is in the case of thick cataract lenses, where the *lenticular* approach is used. Lenticular lenses are really a lens within a lens, the center portion of the lens having refractive power and the marginal portion being a thin cavity allowing the lens to be lighter. Most plastic lenses have greater thicknesses at their edges compared to glass in the case of minus lenses because of plastic's relatively low refractive index. There are now available several "high index" glass and plastic materials available which can eliminate some of the lens thickness.

The main purpose of tinted glasses is to reduce glare. Today there are polarized lenses, and you can use ultraviolet filters like UV 400 to avoid distress and excessive ultraviolet exposure. These lenses can be made with or without tinting. You can buy different types of lenses with different tints to match your outfit.

You may need to have bifocal, trifocal, or multifocal lenses. There are several types from which to choose, depending upon your requirements. For the most part, increased power is placed at the bottom of the lens, since it is normal to look downward when doing close, detailed work. On the other hand, a librarian who needs to see the top rack can have a bifocal near segment placed at the top of the lens instead of at the bottom. Some professionals need the near segment in the middle of the lens. Gradient lenses, without the sharp dividing lines of different power lenses, and called *progressive bifocals*, are available if this is more convenient. Your eye doctor and your dispensing optician (the person who fits your glasses at the optical shop) can assist your selection.

The use of contact lenses has increased in recent years. Because of their great importance, discussion of them is deferred to a special section of this book (Chapter Thirteen).

For an excellent reference about the types of eyeglasses and evaluations of the larger eye chains, see the *Consumer Reports,* August 1993 article, "Glasses," reprinted with permission (Chapter Twelve). This article did a nice comparison of lenses, tints, and frames, and discusses the basics of purchasing eyeglasses. A good rule of thumb is if you currently have a good relationship with an optician who understands your needs and fits you well—stay with him.

Wrap-Up

- "Emmetropia" is the term used to define perfect vision at both distance and near.
- "Hyperopia" is the term used when the image naturally focuses behind the retina. Internal accommodation or focusing may correct hyperopia, allowing younger patients to see well at both distance and near. In some hyperopes, especially older patients, convergent (plus) lenses are needed to correct vision.
- "Myopia" is the term used for a condition in which you can see at near but require an optical device to see at a distance.
- In "astigmatism," the cornea or internal lens are such that two different refractive powers are required to eliminate your distortion.

- In 1993, a reported 24.8 million individuals wore contact lenses and 60 percent of all Americans (approximately 153 million) required some form of vision correction. There were 89 million pairs of vision correction dispensed, including contact lenses. (This information was provided by the 20/20 Optical Group Data Base).

- Approximately 40 million individuals living in the U. S. require eyeglasses for reading.

- Higher index materials allow thick lenses to be thinner.

- The new "flexible frames" are excellent because they are lighter, stronger, and more durable.

- The National Society to Prevent Blindness has estimated that more than 2.4 million eye injuries occur each year. Occupational hazards are more likely in adults, while sports-related injuries are more likely in children and teenagers.

- The lens material of choice is polycarbonate in both non-prescription and prescription eyeglasses. A 2mm center thickness is recommended for street wear, and 3mm for occupational and sports wear. These protection devices are designed to reduce your chances of injury to an acceptable or much lower risk, and should not be perceived as being 100 percent effective in preventing injuries.

Chapter Five

Cataracts and Their Treatment

Warren D. Cross and Lawrence Lynn

Until recently, the clouding of the eye lens—cataracts—were the bane of humankind, causing blindness in all races, primarily affecting the elderly. Fortunately, this situation has vastly improved. Cataracts can be removed easily and painlessly. After cataract removal, an intraocular lens (IOL) can be inserted into the eye and positioned on the same fibers which held the natural lens prior to the IOL implant.

The clouding of the natural lens is now better understood. When blood circulates through the body's arteries and veins, it carries away the body's dead-cell material. The lens is a different matter. It lies within a capsule, like a tiny, sealed football. The lens itself is inside the eyeball, which is also a totally sealed structure. While the lens is developing in utero, the lens nutrients are supplied by an artery and a vein called the *hyaloid system*. Once the lens is fully developed, this "umbilical cord" to the lens atrophies and detaches. The mature lens does not have a direct blood supply and its cells must receive fluid and nutrients through osmosis. Like all organs of the body, the lens must continue to grow and develop. It "grows" by adding long, thin cells to its surface, and burying older lens cells below the surface—sort of a lamination process. What results is a continual slight thickening of the lens.

After forty years or so, the innermost cells of the lens become moderately dehydrated and less flexible. By then, the total volume of the lens may have increased significantly and experienced metabolic changes. The cells in the center of the lens become less transparent, then translucent, then opaque. This change in the transparency of the lens is what we call a *cataract* (Fig. 5–1). Contrary to general thinking, there are various types of cataracts. However, three types are common. Some cataracts become progressively darker brown or *brunescent,* while others are milky white. Heavy deposits of calcium crystals line the inside capsule of others and are referred to as *posterior subcapsular cataracts* or PSCs. In *nuclear cataracts,* aging changes are present in the central nucleus of the lens.

Cataracts are associated with the aging process, but not exclusively. For example, cataracts may be present at birth or develop quickly in a newborn baby. Cataracts can result from diabetes, eye inflammations like iritis or vitritis, measles, and other common diseases. Cataracts can also develop after an eye injury, through taking steroids, or the abuse of drugs. Electromagnetic radiation is known to induce some cataracts.

Cataracts should be removed only if they interfere with your eyesight. Cataracts are not a disease which can spread. Generally, a cataract is harmless to your eye, and merely a nuisance.

Are cataracts preventable? To an extent. Vaccinations hinder the likelihood of suffering infectious diseases, which encourage the development of cataracts, and limiting cataract-producing medication and alcohol ingestion also decreases the likelihood. Antioxidants, especially vitamins E and C and aspirin, may slow cataract growth. Avoiding exposure to ultraviolet radiation will also discourage cataract development. Prescription glasses can be coated with UV 400 films; the non-prescription sunglasses you can buy in a drugstore usually are labeled with their degree of UV protection and should be used outdoors.

There are several types of cataract extractions being performed today. Some ophthalmologists still remove the entire lens in the

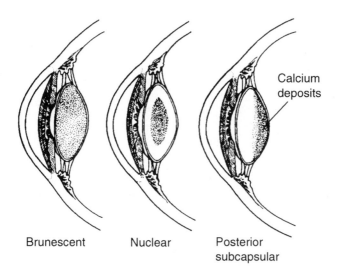

Figure 5–1   Showing various types of cataracts in a lens: left is a brunescent cataract, middle is a nuclear cataract, right is a posterior subcapsular cataract.

capsule, in an operation referred to as *intracapsular cataract extraction*. In this technique you must wait until your lens is "ripe." After a local anesthetic, a tiny incision is made on top of the cornea. A special enzyme is injected into the anterior chamber, which dissolves the ligaments that hold the lens in place. The complete lens in its capsule is then removed with a special loop or forcep. If no replacement lens is implanted, the patient will need thick "Coke bottle" cataract glasses after surgery. A variation of this surgery was invented in Poland and developed in the American clinic founded by Charles Kelman. This procedure, *cryosurgical extraction,* freezes the capsule and lens prior to removal.

Problems have arisen with this approach because it involves a major alteration of the eye's structure. When the lens and capsular bag are removed, the aqueous fluid in the front chamber and the vitreous fluid in the back chamber are now able to move back and forth through the pupil, an unnatural condition. There is an increased incidence of retinal detachment associated with broken lens zonules during surgery and increased vitreous movement after surgery when removing the entire lens. Other possible problems are corneal injuries, glaucoma, a swelling of the macular area in the retina called cystoid macular edema (CME), hemorrhages, and loss of the vitreous fluid from the eye.

Another, more popular procedure is planned *extracapsular extraction*. In this procedure, an incision is made at the surgical limbus, the cornea is tilted forward, and the front surface of the cataract is incised open. The contents of the lens capsule are then removed, the lens capsule is polished, and an intraocular lens is implanted. The great advantage of this type of surgery is that because the zonules and the posterior capsule remain intact, the structural integrity of the eye is retained. The aqueous fluid stays in the front and the vitreous fluid stays in the back of the eye.

The third approach, developed by Dr. Charles Kelman, is called *phacoemulsification,* which is a type of extracapsular cataract extraction. In this procedure, a much smaller corneal incision is made, and the front of the lens capsule is delicately opened (Fig. 5–2A). A phacoemulsification tip is then inserted into the nucleus of the lens (Fig. 5–2B). A titanium needle vibrating at 40,000 times per second breaks up the nucleus of the lens, and the bits of shattered lens are then suctioned out through the probe (Fig. 5–2C). The rear capsule wall is left entirely intact, and is polished to remove any remains of the cataract which could grow and cause a cloudy capsule (Fig. 5–2D).

The intraocular lens is then inserted into the posterior capsule and positioned into place (Fig. 5–2E, Fig. 5–2F). These intraocular replacement lenses are made of different materials and in varying powers from about +2.0 diopters to +30.0 diopters.

Intraocular lens insertion after cataract surgery is commonplace today. These lenses are small single power lenses making a wide range of vision correction possible (Fig. 5–3). Bifocal lens implants are under experimentation, but have not yet been perfected to the point of successful routine FDA-approved implantation.

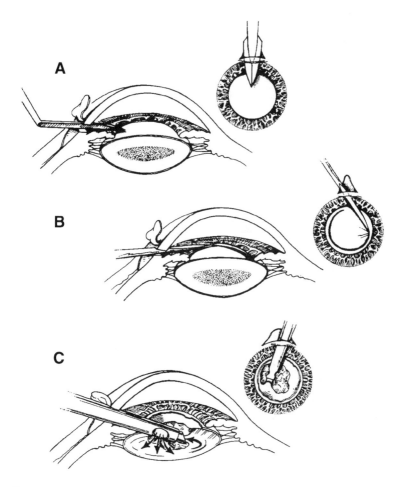

Figure 5–2 Steps in small incision phacoemulsification.
(A) Shows the small incision being made in the surgical limbus toward the top of the cornea.
(B) Shows the front wall (anterior capsule) of the lens being opened gently to permit access to the lens cortex and nucleus.
(C) Shows the phacoemulsification instrument inserted into the patient's actual crystalline lens nucleus and aspirating out the cataractous contents.

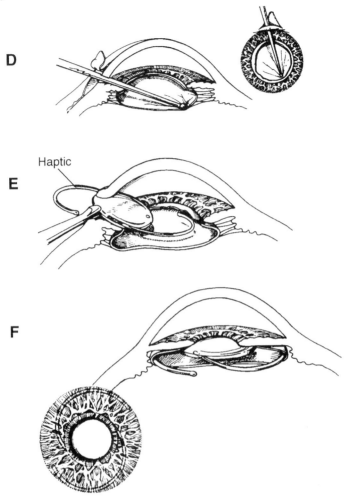

Figure 5-2 *Continued*
(D) Shows the rear wall (posterior capsule) of the lens being cleaned and polished after lens removal to help avoid future opacification or clouding of the posterior capsule.
(E) Shows the new synthetic intraocular lens (IOL) implant being moved into place inside the capsular bag.
(F) Shows the new intraocular lens in place.

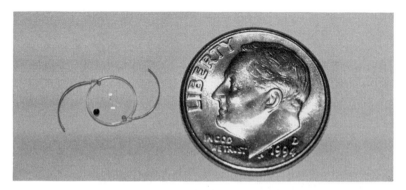

Figure 5–3 The intraocular lens showing its tiny legs called "haptics," which adhere to the patient's tissue. Compare its small size to the ten-cent coin.

Recently, the FDA has approved, for investigational study, a laser machine to remove cataracts. The laser using a small fiberoptic strand is inserted into the cataract using photochemical energy as described in Chapter Six. The altered lens material is irrigated out through a small irrigation/suction tube. Should this machine prove to be effective in the safe removal of cataracts, it will not be available for several years.

There is a 50/50 chance that your vision may decrease gradually after surgery due to a cloudy capsule, which is commonly referred to as a *secondary cataract*. They are easily treated by painless laser "touch up" surgery, referred to as a *YAG posterior capsulotomy*, in the ophthalmologist's office, or in an outpatient clinic. This procedure usually takes less than five to 10 minutes. Since it may take a couple of months to several years for this "membrane" to develop, if it develops at all, the need for a secondary treatment cannot be determined right after primary cataract extraction. The development of this hazy membrane does not mean your ophthalmologist made a mistake, or left some of your cataract in your eye. Rather, it suggests your eye is healthy enough to attempt to grow a new lens. Generally, the younger and healthier you are at the time of your surgery, the more likely you will need a YAG laser (the posterior capsule opened). At age 55, your chances are 50/50 that you will need a YAG laser. Your chances decrease with age.

A commonly asked question is, "What if I have already had a cataract operation but they did not implant an intraocular lens (IOL)? Why don't I have one? Can this be fixed?" Yes, it can. Secondary intraocular lens implantation is the term describing the process of implanting a lens in an eye that had a previous cataract removal. The lens may be placed in front of the iris (colored part of eye) or sutured in place behind the pupil. If you are considering this procedure, you should first try wearing contact lenses.

With the aid of ultrasonic measuring devices and computers, the correct intraocular lens power can be precisely determined with 99 percent accuracy. According to your preference, your post-op sight can be adjusted for seeing at distance in both eyes, or for seeing at near in both eyes, or slightly farsighted in one eye and slightly nearsighted in the other eye. Patients in this last group generally do not need glasses except for driving or detail work, such as reading the newspaper and the telephone book. You need to decide which of these three combinations you wish and discuss them with your surgeon.

Today, eye surgery is astonishingly quick and effective. To avoid problems with anesthesia, you must not eat or drink anything after midnight on the evening before your surgery, unless otherwise instructed by your doctor. Before your surgery, your vital signs are checked, including blood pressure and pulse. A sedative is frequently given, either by mouth or intravenously, early on the morning of surgery to calm your nervousness, if necessary. Then, the anesthetic and antibiotic drops are placed in the eye on which the surgery is to be performed.

Following an almost painless anesthetic injection into the fatty tissues around the eye, you will be taken into surgery. In some centers, selected patients are now adequately anesthetized with topical anesthetic eyedrops only. The upper eyelid is secured, and within minutes the eye operation begins. Following surgery, antibiotic drops or ointment are instilled into the eye to reduce the chance of infection. Cotton gauze and a protective lightweight eye shield are taped in place for protection (Fig. 5–4) after surgery.

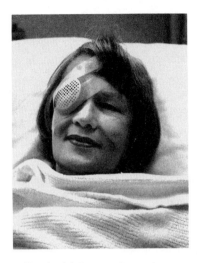

Figure 5–4   A metallic shield frequently used to protect the post-operative eye external to the cotton placed over the closed eye.

In most cases, you are in and out of the outpatient clinic or Ambulatory Surgical Center (ASC) in under three hours. Overnight hospitalization is extremely uncommon. You should not drive immediately after the operation and should spend the afternoon resting. Legal decisions and contracts should not be executed for 24 hours after surgery, due to the lingering influence of the surgery's anesthetics.

A clinic or ASC generally has a licensed anesthesiologist or certified nurse/anesthetist because of the extreme importance of monitoring you and safely preventing movement during surgery. The reason is obvious. In an appendectomy, if the patient moves slightly it can cause minor problems. If a podiatrist was operating on your big toe and it moved slightly, again it would create only a nuisance. But if an eye patient moves after the surgeon has opened the cornea and lens, it could produce a catastrophe, possibly blinding the patient.

Following surgery the eye must not, under any circumstances, be touched or rubbed. This is especially important if you have a "no stitch" procedure. If the eye begins to itch, becomes red or painful, or the vision suddenly becomes worse, the surgeon should immediately re-examine it. While healing, the eye is very delicate and the slightest thing could detach or move the intraocular lens implant or cause the wound to leak. Because most people rub their eyes occasionally during sleep and upon awakening, the eye-shield should be reattached at night or during sleep and taped securely. The patient should be especially careful around small children or pets which might impetuously reach out and touch the eye. Crowds should be avoided for the same reason.

Antibiotic and anti-inflammatory drops usually will be supplied or prescribed by the ophthalmologist for frequent application during the first few days after surgery, then in decreased amounts for a longer period. The clinic may also provide a sterile eyewash for light irrigation and cleaning of the upper and lower eyelids at regular intervals.

For convenience or as a part of your health care plan, your surgical follow up care may be "co-managed" by an optometrist (see Chapter Eighteen).

The upper eyelid may not lift properly right after surgery, giving a droopy-eyed appearance. The eye usually returns to normal within a week or so. It is important for you to avoid bending down, lifting heavy objects, or pushing forcefully forward for several weeks (preferably three weeks). This avoids producing muscular strains, which might increase the fluid pressure within the eye and rupture a healing incision.

Once the shield is removed, the eye may be sensitive and, if so, should be shielded from bright sunlight by sunglasses. It will take from one to two months for the eye to stabilize. At this point, patients who needed glasses for 20/200 vision before surgery may have 20/25 or 20/40 vision. Glasses may not be needed at all, especially in younger patients.

How successful is cataract surgery utilizing procedures such as these? The success rate in patients opting for cataract surgery is listed below. For example, Dr. James Gills, at the St. Luke's

Cataract and Intraocular Lens Institute in Florida, researched thousands of cataract surgeries, and the statistics proved that patients could expect:

99.7 percent chance of better vision.
97.0 percent chance of vision better than 20/40.
90.0 percent chance of vision better than 20/25.
0.01 percent chance of complications leading to blindness.
0.00003 percent chance of complications leading to death.

Therefore, cataract surgery is probably the most successful form of major surgery in existence.

Wrap-Up

- The overall mortality risk of patients undergoing eye surgery has been estimated at 0.06 to 0.18 per 100,000. This level of mortality would be considered a "low but increased risk" surgery. Virtually all deaths were due to pre-existing or patient related factors, such as poor cardiac status or brittle diabetes, not procedure-related factors.
- Cataracts are a natural result of body aging and do not harm the eye, in most cases, if not removed.
- The indications for cataract removal are the cessation or limiting of your activities, such as reading, driving, skiing, and watching television because of your visual impairment.
- The current U. S. government minimum requirement for cataract removal is that your vision be 20/50 or worse.
- The combination of intraocular lens implantation, wound placement, and corneal relaxing incisions allows almost perfect vision in 95–plus percent of those who have had cataract surgery.
- Approximately 500,000 cataract surgeries are performed in the U. S. each year.

- The best cataract surgery procedure is a form of planned extracapsular cataract extraction because the posterior capsule is left intact, helping to stabilize the eye.
- If you are 55 years "young," statistically you have a 50 percent chance that you will require a YAG laser after a cataract removal. The need for YAG laser decreases markedly in older, less healthy patients. The need for YAG laser increases in younger, healthier patients.

Chapter Six

Lasers and Electromagnetic Energy and Eye Surgery

Warren D. Cross

Imagine tree leaves on a sunny day. Besides being beautiful, they are performing the miracle of photosynthesis, making sugars and releasing gases essential to the current composition of the atmosphere. The leaves are adapted to withstanding several hours' dosage of the solar radiation we call sunlight, which makes it to the earth's surface each day. They catch up on regenerating damaged tissue overnight when the earth's rotation carries them into its shadow.

Such is the normal pattern. To help you understand lasers, suppose you take a magnifying glass and focus solar radiation at a small spot on a leaf. You quickly will see a dramatic form of electromagnetic photo activity: heat, fire, and sublimation into soot and ashes. It does not happen ordinarily in nature unless drought lowers the resistance of drying leaves to the point where spontaneous combustion can occur.

Suppose we shine the sunlight through a prism, separating out the wavelengths. To our eyes, they are visible as colors. Because sunlight is composed of all the colors of light with many different frequencies, it is not a pure radiation source. Suppose that now we shine the bright sunlight through a prism. It would enable you to separate the white light into various colors. If we then separated each color, purified it, and intensified the light, it would produce a laser. Each color has its own absorption and photochemical effect. It has been found that artificially produced, intense beams of radiation can be made to do a number of useful things. "Laser" is the acronym derived from *L*ight *A*mplification by *S*timulated *E*mission of *R*adiation. Lasers are beams of radiant energy produced by gases, special crystals, or dyes which, when stimulated by high voltage electricity, emit a stream of energy particles called *photons*. Lasers of distinct wavelengths have different work applications.

Radiation therapy machines, X-ray tubes, microwave ovens, and television transmitters are all special electronic systems designed to generate high-powered, pure electromagnetic radiation. One wavelength can kill cancer, another can help photograph the bones in a broken arm; still another can warm your coffee or bring you the evening news (Table 6–1). The longer the wavelength, the less energy and vice versa. Exposure to any of these radiations will cause mild to fatal damage to living tissue, depending upon intensity and duration of exposure. This is true for nuclear fallout or for X-rays, or for standing around in the sun on a clear day at the beach.

Lifespans have been increased greatly through advances in modern medicine and hygiene. We are living long enough now for environmental influences, like chemicals released into the atmosphere as the byproducts of industry, to have an effect on health. The infectious diseases are in retreat, but in their place are the problems of general bodily decline and the time for cellular dysfunction to kill us.

The building problem is cancer. Cancer is a process whereby cells go crazy and use up the body's resources by making tissue that is neither needed nor helpful. Cancer cannot be cured, but sometimes it can be held at bay. More and more people are being treated for cancer through radiation therapy, often from a beam source. Radiation interferes with DNA synthesis in cells, and can dramatically slow down cell multiplication. Conceptually, the most active cells are affected the most; hopefully that means the tumor.

WAVE LENGTH	NAME	LASER/ ELECTROMAGNETIC FORCE	
6/1,000,000 M 0.006 nanometer	Gamma	Radiation therapy Cancer treatment Radiation Retinopathy	INVISIBLE IONIZING
1/1,000 meter	X-rays		
1/3 meter	Ultraviolet	Photochemical injury Excimer laser Welder's burn UV maculopathy Solar retinopathy	RADIATION
1/2 meter 3/4 meter	Visible light	Photocoagulation argon Blue argon Green krypton Red	
1 meter		Photodisruptive YAG laser	
10 meters 100 meters	Infrared	Thermal effect Carbon dioxide laser	THERMAL
3,000 meters	Microwaves Television FM radio Short-wave Radio AM radio		

Table 6–1 Electromagnetic energy spectrum and its effects on tissue.

Your eye has two cell types which are very active and very sensitive to radiation. The epithelial cells on the front surface of the eye are the most common normal cells that respond readily to radiation, especially ultraviolet (UV). High doses of UV produces the type of burn sailors develop on the water in bright sunlight or the type of burn associated with welding. Prevention of epithelial burning means using glasses or goggles to filter out the dangerous wavelengths.

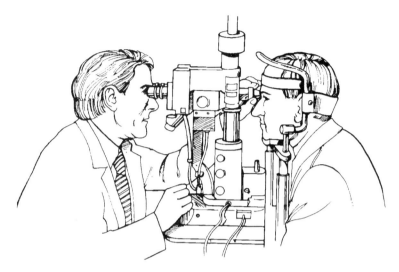

Figure 6–1 Typical argon laser clinical unit for eye surgery.

The cells lining the capillaries in the eye are also very susceptible to radiation damage. This vascular injury of radiation may show up after years, or after only a few days. Damaged vessels begin to leak fluid, the retina swells, the vessels fibrose, and vision dims. Severe problems with the optic nerve can also develop.

On the other hand, the controlled use of radiant energy as lasers has become of enormous help to surgeons, particularly ophthalmologists. The tissue/laser interaction resulting from the argon or the krypton laser is termed "photocoagulation." When the focused laser beam hits a pigmented or dark tissue, an immediate characteristic color change occurs. The proteins are coagulated or denatured similar to cooking an egg until "lightly over." Longer, higher doses can produce vaporization or carbonization of the tissue.

The argon laser is the one most widely used in eye surgery (Fig. 6–1). This "hot" laser's beam is in the visible spectrum, blue or green in color. It is primarily used to seal, or "weld" retinal holes, to seal or cauterize abnormal blood vessels, or to make peripheral iridotomy holes in the iris (as shown in Fig. 6–2). Another valuable use is for glaucoma surgery, as in argon laser trabeculoplasty (ALT).

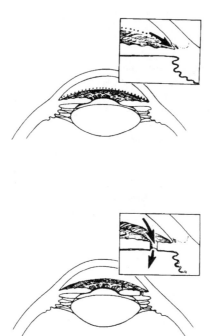

Figure 6–2   Shows the path created by a laser iridotomy.

There are other hot lasers. The argon laser's first cousin is the krypton laser, red in color to human eyes, which is also a thermal laser. It is used generally to treat disease around the macula. The carbon dioxide laser is a thermal laser in the infrared wavelength range. This is a very hot laser capable of cutting almost anything. Because it is so hot, it has less use in ophthalmology than in other areas of medicine.

The YAG neodydium laser is a photo-disruptive laser. It is a "cold laser," an important distinction because if a blood vessel is hit, it will bleed. A YAG will not cauterize a bleeding vessel like an argon laser. In this case, two laser beams invisible to the human eye are carefully focused so that they intersect. At the intersection point, ions and electrons are pulled off the tissue's molecules at sonic speed, producing a rapidly exploding gas bubble or "sonic shock wave." The shockwave mechanically blows tissue apart with a force a mil-

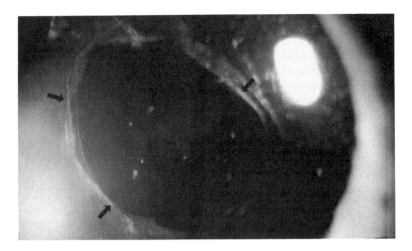

Figure 6–3   Shows the eye after a YAG capsulotomy has been performed.

lion times greater than the atom bomb. Fortunately, the intersection point of the two beams is very small! This laser is used for such jobs as cutting scar tissue or fibrous bands, opening opaque posterior capsules after cataract surgery and making peripheral iridotomies (Fig. 6–3).

The excimer laser (short for *EXCI*ted Di*MER*) is an ionizing laser, meaning that it strips electrons from the molecules of the target tissue (Fig. 6–4). This is a very precise "cold laser" beam which cuts at the molecular level. Inert gases, such as argon and fluoride, or xenon and chloride, are bound together by a high-voltage electrical field. When the current stops, an ultraviolet photon shorter than visual light is emitted, producing photoablation.

This laser generates an ultraviolet photon with twice the energy of the carbon-carbon bonds that hold our body together. When our bonds are struck by this high-energy particle, they break apart. In Table 6–1, you will notice that this is also a photochemical laser. In photochemical lasers, the injury to the tissue is a form of light damage that is a consequence of a certain biochemical reaction. This produces a degeneration of tissue without temperature elevation. The small carbon chains go out into space. This is a very precise "cold laser" beam capable of essentially cutting at the molecular

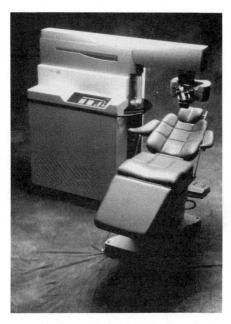

Figure 6–4   The excimer laser. (Photograph contributed by Summit Technology.)

level; a "molecular knife," so to speak. In eye surgery, the tissue degenerates without temperature elevation, creating an excellent device with which to reshape the cornea.

Lasers are particularly useful as ophthalmic tools. Time spent in surgery and recovery have been sharply reduced by them; the surgeon also can operate with greater accuracy and safety. In 1991 the *Ocular Surgery News* reported that over 80 percent of ophthalmologists were using argon lasers for iridotomies. Nearly 90 percent now use the YAG laser to treat secondary cataracts.

Lasers allow treatments that are safe, fast, and less likely to cause infections. Millions of dollars are being spent annually on evaluating and testing lasers to improve the future of our vision.

More about how, when, and why these lasers are used is described in the previous and following chapters which discuss the specific diseases and problems of the eye requiring laser treatment (Chapters Five, Seven, Nine, Eleven).

Wrap-Up

- Laser is an acronym derived from *L*ight *A*mplification by *S*timulated *E*mission of *R*adiation.
- Electromagnetic energy wavelengths begin at approximately one-billionth of a meter long to several miles long.
- The visible light humans see is E.M.E. with wavelengths of approximately one-half to one meter in length.
- Lasers, television stations, X-ray machines, and light bulbs are all specialized electrical devices capable of generating relatively uniform wavelength E.M.E.
- Lasers of different wavelengths have different characteristics and applications.
- The argon laser is the most common laser in ophthalmology. It is a "thermal laser" and is useful for "welding," cutting and cauterizing.
- The YAG laser is an example of a "cool" photodisruptive laser which is used for cutting.
- The excimer laser, a "molecular knife," is a cold photochemical or photoablation laser capable of cutting at the molecular level without injuring the adjacent tissue by heat or explosions.
- Properly understood and used, E.M.E. can become very beneficial to man instead of injurious and lethal.

Chapter Seven

Glaucoma

Lawrence Lynn and Warren D. Cross

Nature and Diagnosis

"Glaucoma" is a general term for several eye conditions in which the intraocular pressure (IOP) of fluids within the eye is higher than normal. This is similar to high blood pressure in the eye. High intraocular pressure can destroy the eye's delicate arteries, veins, and nerve fibers. If IOP builds up, the optic nerve at the back of the eye may atrophy, causing vision to become incomplete, fuzzy, or just dim. If left untreated, matters can reach the point where progressive loss of peripheral vision, even total blindness, can occur.

Glaucoma is a serious matter. Without the full range of peripheral vision, the operation of an automobile or any other mobile equipment becomes very dangerous. In fact, a large but virtually unrecognized number of accidents happen each year simply because someone in a vehicle couldn't see a hazard well enough or quickly enough to avoid an accident. Millions of Americans are driving around on our highways with a reduced visual field, endangering themselves and those they may hit. The early detection and treatment of glaucoma could help reduce this problem. (Fig. 7–1.)

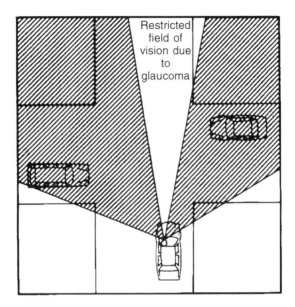

Figure 7–1 Sketch depicting severe limitation of the visual field, or "tunnel vision," of a patient suffering from glaucoma. Note the impossibility for the driver to see the cars coming toward the intersection from either direction.

Diagnosing Glaucoma vs. "Glaucoma Suspect"

There are certain people who have elevated intraocular pressure measurements on multiple checkups, but who do not develop the progressive anatomical and visual changes characteristic of glaucoma. These patients are followed closely and are diagnosed as *glaucoma suspect* or as *ocular hypertensives.*

Making the distinction between glaucoma suspect and true glaucoma is not always easy. A number of factors other than elevated IOPs on multiple checkups are involved in diagnosing glaucoma. These include a family history of glaucoma, visual field defects, and optic nerve changes characteristic of glaucoma. True glaucoma is usually an inherited trait. If you have relatives who have glaucoma, you should be checked regularly. Early diagnosis of glaucoma significantly increases the likelihood of successful treatment. The best way to prevent glaucoma injury is to be tested every year or two after the age of 40 to see whether or not your IOP is elevated.

Our eyes are designed to operate in a state of pressure balance maintained by internal fluids resisting the atmospheric weight outside. Normal intraocular pressure averages 21 mm Hg or less, starting slightly higher early in the morning and declining due to body hormonal changes as the day proceeds. Pressure between 22 mm Hg and 28 mm Hg is suspicious of glaucoma, and IOP higher than 28 mm Hg may indicate glaucoma. Sometimes the pressure is high enough that a specialist can tell simply by feeling the eyeball through the eyelid. A normal eye feels slightly bouncy and rubbery, like a tennis ball. An eye with moderate to severe glaucoma can feel as hard as a rock.

The best way to identify and follow glaucoma is through the examination of the pale-colored central area of the optic nerve, which is commonly referred to as the "optic cup." The optic cup is where the optic nerve fibers in the retina merge to become the optic nerve. The optic cup is usually shallow and about one-quarter of the optic nerve's diameter. In glaucoma, the cup is forced into a deep "bean pot" shape with bloated sides. The retinal vessels located in the center of the optic nerve become displaced to the sides of the optic nerve, and in severe cases, their origin may not even be visible.

Another way to identify and follow glaucoma is to examine the filtering angle with a gonio lens. The gonio lens is a contact lens with small mirrors at various angles through which interior structures of the eye can be examined under high magnification.

Finally, you may be given a visual field test. Optic nerve damage first affects the peripheral vision. Glaucoma can cause a narrow field of vision and/or enlargement of the normal blind spot which can affect your functional vision. In most cases, the enlargement of the blind spot is not noticed by the patient. Most examiners are reluctant to diagnose glaucoma unless there are positive results found in nearly all of these factors, and at least several elevated IOP measurements.

Chronic Open-Angle Glaucoma (COAG)

To fully understand the several different types of glaucoma, let's discuss briefly the fluids of the eye (Fig. 7–2A).

The aqueous humor is continually secreted by the ciliary processes which are located directly behind the peripheral margin of the iris. The aqueous humor circulates through the front chamber of the eye, providing water and nutrients to the cornea and the lens. The aqueous humor then flows into the rear chamber of the eye, through the pupil, and then returns to the front chamber of the eye. Finally, the aqueous humor filters through the trabecular meshwork which is located at the extreme edge of the eye's iris, through the canal of Schlemm and into adjacent blood vessels where it is dispersed through the blood system.

In most glaucoma patients, the trabecular meshwork becomes less permeable. When this happens, the aqueous is unable to adequately drain from the eye in the normal pressure ranges. Since the aqueous continually rejuvenates itself, IOP rises. Less commonly, pressure increases occur when there is an increase in the rate of formation of aqueous. Whatever the origin, glaucoma can gradually creep up without causing pain or much sense of changed eyesight. This usually occurs after age 40. Males and females experience glaucoma in equal proportion. Treatment involves trying to reduce the rate of aqueous formation, or unclogging the filtration network.

Deterioration of peripheral vision is hard for you to detect unless severe changes develop. This type of glaucoma, which is usually irreversible, is referred to as *chronic open-angle glaucoma* (COAG), or *open-angle glaucoma.* COAG occurs in two to three percent of the population and is approximately 10 times more common than other types of glaucoma. It is found four to five times more often in African-American patients than in Caucasian patients. In the United States, COAG is the most frequent cause of blindness among African-Americans and the second most frequent cause of blindness among Caucasians.

Low-Tension Glaucoma

One curious version of open-angle glaucoma is "normal tension glaucoma," sometimes referred to as "low-tension glaucoma." As the name implies, this is an eye condition which causes gradual optic nerve atrophy and the same visual field defects as in progressive

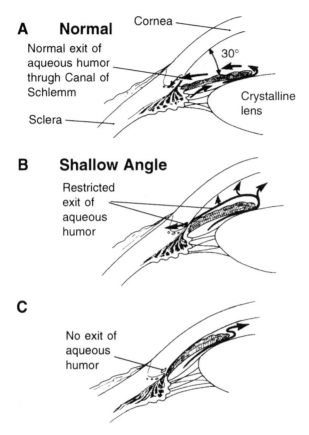

Figure 7–2 (A) The angle structure in a healthy eye. Note the arrow-marked path of the aqueous humor from its source in the ciliary processes, past the iris, through the pupil into the anterior chamber and its departure from the eye through the trabecular meshwork and canal of Schlemm.
(B) Compare this shallow angle structure to the normal angle in Fig. 7–2A. The shallowness causes a great probability of adhesion of the iris to the cornea. It portends a danger of closed-angle glaucoma.
(C) In this drawing of acute closed-angle glaucoma, the iris has become compressed against the cornea. Exit of aqueous humor is impossible. This condition should be treated immediately.

chronic open-angle glaucoma. The differences are the angles are open and IOPs are almost normal or sometimes less than normal. Approximately 20 percent of all open-angle glaucomas fall into this group. There are no convincing theories about what causes this malady, and neither medical management nor surgeries have been effective in predictably reversing or stopping it.

Acute-Angle Closure Glaucoma (CAG)

Considerably less frequent than COAG is the potentially catastrophic condition of *closed-angle glaucoma,* (CAG) also called *acute congestive glaucoma* or *primary angle closure glaucoma.* This condition tends to occur in people who have, as part of their genetic inheritance, eyes with a narrower angle structure (Fig. 7–2B). These potentially glaucomatous eyes are generally smaller than normal and have a narrower, smaller front chamber. This usually occurs in older patients in which the lens is usually proportionately larger than normal, tending to push the iris forward, further narrowing the angle. If the shallow angle becomes clogged, or the peripheral iris at its base is pressed tightly against the cornea, it becomes impossible for the aqueous humor to flow through the trabecular meshwork and exit the eye (Fig. 7–2C). The IOP increases rapidly, producing unbearable pain, extreme nausea, hazy vision, intense vomiting, and general weakness—an emergency situation. Because these symptoms can be easily confused with those produced by a stroke, they can be misdiagnosed unless a doctor recognizes the closure of the angle structure, haziness of the cornea, injection of the sclera, and the stationary mid-dilated pupil. Acute closed-angle glaucoma will rapidly result in damage to the retina and the optic nerve, and can result in blindness if not treated immediately.

Closed-angle glaucoma can, in certain cases, be accompanied by the growth of tiny adhesions called *synechiae* on the iris. These synechiae seem to "weld" the marginal area of the iris and cornea together, blocking drainage through the trabecular meshwork. Synechiae begin to form as quickly as 12 hours after the onset of closed-angle glaucoma.

"Secondary" and Other Causes of Glaucoma

While nearly all glaucomas have their roots in inheritance, some are caused by some other medical problems. When this happens they are called "secondary glaucomas." They can be temporary and innocuous while other types are quite serious and difficult to treat. A cataract can occasionally cause glaucoma. If the cataractous lens is permitted to continue growing until it pushes the iris forward, it can cause obstruction of the aqueous flow. A tumor, benign or malignant, may develop in the eye. If a tumor develops, it may cause inflammation or push the iris out of shape, blocking the angle.

Diabetes, through its effects on the veins and arteries, can cause a secondary glaucoma. Uveitis, a severe and unfortunately quite frequent inflammation of the uvea—the iris, ciliary body, vitreous, choroid, and retina—can cause swelling of tissues and increased viscosity of the aqueous inside the eye, and through this lead to secondary glaucoma. When blunt trauma to the eye causes a rupture or tearing of the filtering angle with bleeding into the edge, *traumatic glaucoma,* or *angle-recession glaucoma,* may develop at any time because of the injury.

Glaucoma can occur in a growing fetus when an abnormal excess tissue forms, obstructing the trabeculae and flow of the aqueous humor. If not surgically corrected, the result, although rare, can cause abnormal enlargement of the baby's eye, which is referred to as *buphthalmos* ("ox-eye").

Treatment for Chronic Open-Angle Glaucoma

The early treatment of open-angle glaucoma is critical because the damage caused to the eye is irreversible. A glaucoma treatment plan must be vigorously adhered to once started. There are plenty of stories about patients who, for one misguided reason or another, stopped using their glaucoma medications and stopped returning to the doctor for their glaucoma checkup visits. Some manage to make themselves irreversibly blind in the process.

Usually the medications are short-acting eyedrops which must be applied two to four times a day. It is recommended that patients allow at least five minutes between the application of different eyedrops. The eye can only hold a maximum of two eyedrops, and the second eyedrop will probably wash the first one out of the eye.

Because COAG is such a slowly developing problem, it gives the doctor and the patient time to explore various approaches in the treatment. Most patients are usually started on low dose beta-blockers such as Timoptic™, Betoptic S™, and Betagan™ taken once a day. If the eyedrops fail to control the glaucoma, the frequency and dosage are increased to twice a day. If you have a history of cardiac problems and pulmonary asthmatic conditions, these conditions could be exacerbated by the beta-blockers, and therefore, may not be advised. Other medications prescribed may be miotics or epinephrine-related drugs such as Propine™. Propine™ is the most frequently used because it has very little cardiac or pulmonary effect, although it may cause a slight rise in heart-rate and blood pressure. Some patients develop a sensitivity to Propine™ in the form of persistently red eyes, which may become uncomfortable. When Propine™ is used in combination with a beta-blocker, each drug's effects are significantly enhanced.

Pilocarpines are very well-established drugs that are remarkably safe and useful for the treatment of glaucoma. They are being used less frequently because these drugs metabolize in six hours. So, to be most effective they must be used four times per day. A more convenient, longer-acting four percent pilocarpine gel may be used at bedtime. Pilocarpine is a miotic drug which makes your pupil smaller. This "snake eye pupil" may produce a problem in night vision, especially for those who have cataracts. Pilocarpine also has the bothersome characteristic of stimulating accommodation (as if you were focusing at near) causing temporary nearsightedness. Pilocarpine burns when instilled into the eye, which may make it difficult for you to stay enthusiastic about using it four times a day.

In moderately severe cases of glaucoma, longer-acting medications such as anticholinesterases (Floropryl™, Humorsol™, Phospholine Iodide™), or epinephrine (Propine™) may be prescribed alone or in conjunction with other eyedrops. In the more severe cases of glaucoma, oral or intravenous medications, such as carbonic anhydrase inhibitors (Diamox™, Neptazane™, Daranide™, or MZM ™ (methazolamide)) may be used. These medications lower the rate of aqueous humor formation. Sometimes a combination of two or more eyedrops or a combination of eyedrops and oral medication is required to control the glaucoma.

How these drugs act to lower the intraocular pressure is not fully known. If you have a mild glaucoma, particularly if you have fair skin and light colored eyes, medications may keep the glaucoma and IOP under control for long periods, sometimes for your lifetime, without surgery. On the other hand, there are some glaucomas which become progressively worse despite the most comprehensive use of different eyedrops and levels of medicinal treatment (Table 7–1).

If the necessary alternative is surgery, occasionally it will be found that the IOP is so high that the cornea is too cloudy for the laser to effectively penetrate the haze. This means postponing your surgery from one to three days. In an emergency situation, a paracentesis may be performed which usually relieves the pressure immediately. A paracentesis is the painless removal of excess aqueous fluid from the anterior chamber using a very fine knife or needle. An alternative treatment is the use of oral and topical medications which will decrease the intraocular pressure, causing the cornea to clear and thus allowing surgical intervention.

There are several surgical methods to decrease aqueous production which do not involve incisional surgery. Cyclocryotherapy freezes the ciliary body with a probe which circulates liquid nitrogen against the sclera. This controlled freezing destroys the underlying ciliary body and decreases aqueous production. Using laser beams, the YAG trans-scleral cyclophotocoagulator inactivates the ciliary body and permanently destroys the tissue which produces the aqueous humor.

Surgery can also be used to release fluids. Argon laser trabeculoplasty (ALT) is a painless non-incisional laser procedure in which small holes are made in the trabecular meshwork to allow the aqueous humor to easily drain from the anterior

DRUG	SIDE EFFECTS
Betagan™ (Levobunolol HCl)	C—Ocular burning, stinging, red eyelids. R—Decrease in heart rate and blood pressure, dizziness.
Betoptic S™ (Betaxolol HCl)	C—Ocular discomfort, blurred vision. R—Light sensitivity, corneal irritation, decreased heart rate, difficulty breathing.
Daranide™ (Dichlorphenamide)	C—Nausea, vomiting, headache. R—Nervousness, tingling in extremities, weakness.
Diamox™ (Acetazolamide)	C—Tingling in extremities and lips, fatigue, nausea. R—Ringing in ears, drowsiness, confusion, and metallic taste in mouth.
Epifrin™ (Epinephrine)	C—Eye ache, headache, conjunctival redness. R—Allergic lid reaction.
Eppy/N™ (Epinephryl Borate)	C—Headache, palpitations, faintness. R—Macular condition with decreased visual acuity, pigmentary deposits.
Floropryl™ (Isoflurophate)	C—Ocular stinging, burning, tearing, redness. R—Lid twitch, headache, nearsightedness.
Glaucon™ (Epinephrine HCl)	C—Ocular stinging, burning. R—Ocular pigmentation, headache, palpitation.
Humorsol™ (Demecarium Br)	C—Ocular stinging, burning, tearing, redness. R—Lid twitch, headache, nearsightedness.
Iopidine™ (Apraclonidine)	C—Red and itchy eyes, tearing. R—Dry mouth and nose, change of taste.
IsoptoCarbachol™ (Carbachol)	C—Ocular stinging, burning, tearing, redness. R—Lid twitch, headache, nearsightedness, salivation, fainting, cramps, cardiac arrhythmia.
IsoptoCarpine™ (Pilocarpine HCl)	C—Ocular stinging, burning, tearing, redness. R—Lid twitch, headache, nearsightedness.
MZM™ (Methazolamide)	C—Nausea, vomiting, headache. R—Nervousness, tingling in extremities, weakness.

Table 7–1   List of frequently used glaucoma medications.

DRUG	SIDE EFFECTS
Phospholine Iodide™ (Echothiophate)	C—Ocular stinging, burning, tearing, headache. R—Ocular redness, retinal detachment, lid twitch, nearsightedness, iritis, uveitis, cataracts.
Pilagan™ (Pilocarpine Nitrate)	C—Blurred vision, poor dark adaptation. R—Ocular redness, retinal detachment, lens opacities.
Pilocar™ (Pilocarpine HCl)	C—Tearing, headache, redness. R—Ciliary spasm, retinal detachment, nearsightedness, cataract.
Pilopine Gel™ (Pilocarpine HCl)	C—Tearing, redness, burning, headache. R—Ciliary spasm, corneal irritation, retinal detachment.
Propine™ (Dipivefrin HCl)	C—Burning, stinging, conjunctivitis. R—Tachycardia, hypertension, arrhythmia.
Timoptic™ (Timolol Maleate)	C—Headache, bradycardia, depression, dizziness. R—Hypotension, arrhythmia, nausea, fainting, stroke.
Neptazane™ (Methazolamide)	C—Tingling in extremities, fatigue, nausea. R—Ringing in ears, drowsiness, confusion.

C—Common side effect
R—Rare side effect
™ —Trade mark

Table 7-1 *Continued*

chamber. This surgery generally lowers the IOP by 4 mm Hg to 9 mm Hg, and the effect lasts from two to five years. It can generally be repeated twice.

If laser surgery fails to lower IOP to a satisfactory level, it may be necessary to do a "trabeculectomy," which is a surgical filtering procedure. The surgeon mechanically opens the blocked passages in the trabecular meshwork, creating a controlled exit of the aqueous fluid into the surgically created space between the conjunctiva and the sclera where it can be reabsorbed. If a trabeculectomy is not satisfactory, it can be repeated.

In the most severe instances, plastic or silicone tubes with or without pumps are permanently sutured into tiny holes cut through the sclera. The fluid then drains into the subconjunctival space to be reabsorbed into the blood stream.

Treating Acute-Angle Closure Glaucoma (AACG)

Treatment of acute-angle closure glaucoma is usually a completely different scenario because time is of the essence. Immediate efforts are made to reduce your IOP. Such measures include pilocarpine and other eyedrops, oral or intravenous medications. A *peripheral iridotomy* procedure performed with either a YAG or argon laser, or a combination of both, can also provide adequate circulation pathways and reduce the intraocular pressure. If your pressure remains high and your cornea is too hazy for the laser to penetrate, as a last resort paracentesis, or draining, of the anterior chamber provides immediate relief from glaucoma. Later a laser, surgical filtration procedure, or even a cataract extraction may be needed to fully treat your condition.

In some cases of angle-closure glaucoma, a surgical *peripheral iridectomy* may be recommended. After making a tiny incision through the limbus, the surgeon gently grasps the iris near its base and removes a section of the iris. This procedure permits the aqueous to bypass the blockage and relieve pressure.

After acute-angle closure glaucoma has been brought under control, the surgeon may recommend a preventative iridectomy for the opposite eye. If the angles are narrow, there is a 50 percent chance of developing acute-angle glaucoma in the other eye.

Treatment of Congenital Glaucoma

Treatment for congenital glaucoma in very young children may involve removal of the tissue which is blocking the trabecular meshwork. The measurement of IOP in young children is more complicated than in adults because children rarely cooperate for tonometry. A general anesthetic is usually required for tonometry, and gonioscopy is performed to study the angle structure. When general anesthetic is necessary, it is generally performed in a hospital under the constant supervision of anesthesiologists. For adults, glaucomas are usually treatable with local anesthesia in out-patient facilities.

Treatment for Secondary Glaucoma

Treatments for secondary glaucomas are as different as their causes. They may involve a simultaneous cataract extraction. If a tumor is present, whether benign or malignant, its removal is necessary before the glaucoma can be treated. In the case of uveitis, usually the glaucoma must be treated while the inflamed tissue is being treated. Treatment may include an extensive medical evaluation to determine the cause, such as rheumatoid arthritis, sarcoidosis, lupus, and other autoimmune conditions.

After glaucoma treatment, patients frequently ask if there is any danger in using the eyes for normal purposes such as driving, movies, watching television, or reading. The general answer is no.

Complications of Glaucoma Surgery

There are five main potential complications resulting from unsuccessful glaucoma surgery. All are rare.

1. Failure to alleviate high IOP, with post-op IOP remaining at unacceptably high levels. Continued high IOP means further damage to the optic nerve and continued gradual worsening of vision with open-angle glaucoma. The solution to this problem is to repeat the surgery and/or to alter your medications.
2. An infection caused by unwanted bacteria entering the eye during surgery. The patient may feel pain, which can be intense; the eye may become red, and may contain a discharge accompanied by decreasing vision. Antibiotic relief is generally required at a high systemic as well as topical level.

3. Major or minor internal bleeding in the eye. If minor, it will probably resolve itself. If severe, the eye may have to be opened to stop the bleeding and to irrigate the excess blood away from the path of vision.
4. Retinal detachment which may appear as a "falling curtain" or "veil" over a portion of the field of vision.
5. Corneal complications, the most severe of which is injury and loss of the endothelial cells, which compose the innermost layer of the cornea. The endothelial cells are vital and must be preserved in sufficient number and health to avoid corneal translucency or opacity. In extreme cases, corneal grafts may be required.

Once any procedure has been performed, it is vital that post-operatively you follow the steps listed below:

1. Following surgery, use the antibiotic eyedrops and other medications at the frequency suggested by your ophthalmologist.
2. Return for post-operative checkups as advised by your eye doctor. Should a complication occur, such as infection or elevated intraocular pressure, treatment can begin early.
3. Return periodically for further tonometry to make sure that the IOP is under control.
4. Chronic open-angle glaucoma has in all likelihood *not been cured* by medication or surgery. It has been brought under control in order to arrest or defer further damage to the eye. You and your ophthalmologist will have to work together to prevent additional damage.

Wrap-Up

- There are generally four criteria necessary for you to be diagnosed as having "glaucoma." Generally, it means your blood relatives have had glaucoma, your intraocular pressures are above normal (over 21 mm Hg) on several measurements, your "optic cup" is becoming larger and more "bean pot" shaped, and/or your visual fields have been changing in patterns typical of glaucoma.

- A diagnosis of elevated intraocular pressures or "glaucoma suspect" is used in situations where your pressures are higher than normal but no significant changes have occurred in your visual fields or optic nerves.
- Generally speaking, glaucoma can be controlled by eyedrops and occasionally oral medications.
- Laser and/or incisional surgical procedures are still required to control glaucoma in some patients.
- Severe headaches in the area of one eye, blurred vision, "red eye," and possibly nausea are typical signs of an acute attack of angle-closure glaucoma. See your ophthalmologist or go to the closest Emergency Room immediately.
- Most glaucoma treatments will require the use of medications for the remainder of your life.
- COAG, the most common glaucoma, is painless.
- If you have a history of significant eye trauma, such as a fish hook in the eye, a baseball injury, or a racquetball injury, you are more likely to develop "secondary glaucoma" later in your life. You need annual eye examinations.

Chapter Eight

Corneal Refractive Surgery

Warren D. Cross

Refractive surgery is defined as a surgical procedure which alters how the eye focuses light and decreases your dependency on "ophthalmic crutches" such as glasses and contact lenses. Ideally, this would be accomplished to the point of perfect vision both near and far. It may not always be possible at this time to rid you completely of your need for glasses. In this situation, the goal may be to decrease the distortion and imbalance that may be present. High amounts of astigmatism, and large differences in the prescription between your two eyes (anisometropia) may cause you to have trouble reading, walking, climbing stairs, and driving. Fortunately, many procedures are available to help remedy these visual problems.

Refractive Surgery

Part of the decision to permit refractive surgery has to do with what you want to achieve from it. If glasses are not perceived as uncomfortable hindrances, and the bare thought of surgery is terrifying, no amount of argument about the yield of superior eyesight is going to be convincing! For that matter, there are some professions where an avuncular, studious look may seem appropriate, as in the library sciences, banking, or editing.

However, if your work is such that wearing eyeglasses is uncomfortable or impossible, a turn toward surgery may make sense. Any sort of activity which requires a lot of exertion or danger, such as police work, construction, firefighting, or the military would be helped through surgical enhancement of the eye. For that matter, safety around the house is enhanced if you don't have to fumble for glasses or lenses in a tight moment, such as discovering that the kitchen is on fire, or hearing a strange noise in the house.

Here's an exotic example of a work-related need for refractive surgery. My patient, an astronaut who was scheduled for several impending shuttle flights, was becoming progressively nearsighted. Initially, he had been 20/20 without glasses but had become 20/200 without glasses in both eyes and was unable to get along without his glasses. Yet, in the weightless, zero humidity environment of space, neither option would do, nor be permitted. He decided that the only way to keep his astronautical career flying was to have RK (Radial Keratotomy) done. The operation went successfully. He flew three times, and he was able to perform strenuous activities, including stepping outside into space to repair a satellite arm, with absolutely no problems. Without RK, he would have had to turn his position over to someone else and resign himself to earthbound support work. My commercial divers report the same results from 200 feet below sea level. These are the highs and lows of our 14,000 cases to date!

Other good candidates for RK are athletes who can't be bothered with glasses or contacts while swimming, riding a bull, sky diving, or fencing. You don't want to suddenly find yourself minus one eye's sight right in the middle of a basketball game, or calling time to hunt for a third pair of glasses when your team is within striking range of a touchdown. No, to be competitive, you have to be able to see as well as the best, and through the most effective means.

The last major group of individuals, who need to consider refractive surgery, are those who might otherwise have been satisfied to continue using glasses or contact lenses, but no longer can for one reason or another. The elderly may develop a problem in remembering where they put their glasses. After refractive surgery, usually you can lose them for good. Normal aging, anatomical changes, dry eyes, allergies—all can make contact lens use intolerable. Just applying them can become a trial if arthritis or senility come into the picture. After RK, using your eyes means only opening your eyelids each morning.

You can see that the insurance companies, which insist that refractive surgery is cosmetic, probably are more concerned with holding onto operating capital than facing facts. A patient wearing contact lenses looks the same as someone who has had RK. In fact, fewer than five percent of the patients who took part in the Perspective Evaluation of Radial Keratotomy (PERK) study by the federal government had approached refractive surgery for other than functional reasons.

If considering refractive surgery, you will have questions as you begin investigating the various procedures and surgeons. The result of this investigation is usually a lot of diverse opinions either pro or con. Some ophthalmologists are opposed to operating on a "normal" cornea or eye. Other surgeons may minimize the complexity of the surgery and possible complications. The truth lies somewhere in-between. The more care taken in the choice of a surgeon, the more likely you will obtain the desired results.

Most refractive surgeries are "elective." For example, a patient who has been highly nearsighted for 40 years need not rush into a refractive surgical procedure and can approach it slowly and deliberately.

Risks and Surgeon Selection

All surgeries carry a risk factor: from simple surgeries such as the removal of a small mole, to complex eye operations and open heart surgery. Many eye doctors have specific handouts and/or books which aid in understanding the eye procedure you are considering. Video tape and video disc programs explain risk factors and are available in most doctors' offices. It is wise to read the informed consent. If the document is difficult to understand, or is unclear, your doctor should be happy to answer your questions. The surgeon should inform you about possible risk factors and answer any questions regarding risk factors. Your surgeon's experience, training, successful surgeries, types of surgeries, and number of complications encountered should give a good indication of what the odds are that the surgery will be successful. Equally important is, how much does the initial examination and surgery cost? What is the additional cost if an adjustment (or two) is needed, or if a complication occurs? Ninety-five percent of corneal refractive patients see very well with 97 percent showing improvement, but one to three percent are disappointed and may even see worse after surgery. Statistics are never important if you are the patient who does not show improvement. Therefore, it is wise to schedule several consultations before choosing a surgeon. If you still cannot decide which surgeon to use, then ask for three patient names whom you may call to discuss their experiences with surgery, postoperative care, and surgical results. You may also want to ask who actually performed their surgery, who took care of them after their surgery, and if they were happy with their care.

Finally, you must assimilate the impressions and data to determine the "risk, reward, and benefit ratio" of the surgery. If a perfect 20/20 is the only acceptable result, then you probably are not a good surgical candidate. If what you desire is to "improve organ function without glasses or contact lenses" and you understand that perfection is not guaranteed, then select a surgeon from your research and enjoy your improved vision. The result most likely will be goodbye to glasses!

Refractive Surgery Involving Intraocular Lenses

To correct or change your refraction, you must either change your corneal power or change the lens inside your eye. Cataract surgery with an intraocular lens implant removes a hazy lens, and is also an excellent example of refractive surgery where changing the lens is involved. This surgery is one of the most common refractive procedures performed today, and is often forgotten as a refractive procedure. If the cornea and retina are normal, there is a 97 to 99 percent plus success rate for a successful surgery and excellent vision following this procedure.

Research currently under scrutiny involves the insertion of a very thin second lens into the front chamber near the iris without touching or removing your natural lens. A primary concern about this procedure is that an additional lens near the natural clear lens might cause a cataract or glaucoma as time progresses.

A third technique involving the lens is called a *clear lensectomy*, "Ectomy" means "the removal of." The power of the lens in your eye is about plus 20 diopters. In this procedure, your doctor would remove your clear natural lens if your prescription for glasses was in the range of minus 20 to 24 (high myopia). Because of the high risk of retinal detachment, a retinal consult before and after surgery is needed. High myopia is rare, but the surgery works like magic when appropriate. One of my patients, a young married man, had consulted numerous surgeons several years ago in the U.S. and was told he was too nearsighted for correction. His vision was so poor that he could only see an object if it was held two inches or less in front of his eye. He had a minus 21 refractive error in one eye and a minus 23 refractive error in his other eye. The first night after a clear lensectomy was performed, he took his patch off and cried. He could see his wife across the room for the first time, unaided by glasses. His vision after surgery had been corrected without glasses to 20/25 and 20/40 respectively.

Corneal Refractive Surgery

The remaining procedures involve changing the corneal power. The changes made occur by making incisions (RK), sculpting the surface (excimer laser), or by changing layers of tissue in the cornea.

Radial Keratotomy

This is probably the most popular and best-known refractive procedure. This procedure is known by several different names, such as *RK, radial keratoplasty* or *radial keratotomy*. Since this procedure is the most common and also the most controversial refractive procedure, it will be discussed a little more extensively than the others in this chapter.

Dr. Tutomo Sato of Japan initially conceived and performed the procedure in the early 1950s. The function and purpose of endothelial cells were then unknown. Surgical microscopes and the sharp knives of today were also absent. Without these microscopes and knives, Dr. Sato operated on the wrong side of the cornea—the inside. As you might have guessed, 80 percent of the corneas turned opaque. However, about 20 percent of the corneas survived, and their myopia was corrected. With an 80 percent failure rate, Dr. Sato did not have long lines waiting for refractive surgery.

The current procedure began in Russia in the 1970s by Dr. Svyatoslav Fyodorov. RK consists of making a variety of very thin, fine radial incisions through the corneal surface in a variety of patterns around the periphery of the cornea (imagine cutting a pizza, see Fig. 8–1F and Fig. 8–2). Since the cornea in a very nearsighted eye is very steep like a mountain, the purpose of RK is to flatten the center of your cornea.

As the periphery of the cornea is incised, it bulges outward because of the natural pressure of the eye inside. As the periphery "pooches outward," the central area that you see through becomes flatter and therefore less nearsighted. The exact number, pattern and length of incisions is determined by your surgeon, usually with the aid of computer programs and nomograms. Your exact prescription, age, sex, curvature of cornea, corneal thickness, and intraocular pressure are all variables used in planning an individual RK. Many people like this procedure because the central area through which you see is untouched, which is in contrast to other procedures.

In the first weeks following surgery, you will notice temporary but startling variations in your vision. Since overnight the eyelids have been closed, evaporation from the cornea is markedly reduced. Therefore, the cornea is slightly swollen with fluid in the early morning. This phenomenon produces variations into farsightedness. The fuzziness clears with normal surface evaporation from the cornea. You will also notice starburst, halo, and glare effects while healing of the tiny cuts is underway. Just about all of these surprise changes in vision are gone within a couple of weeks, but in some cases they can linger on for as much as a year while gradually getting

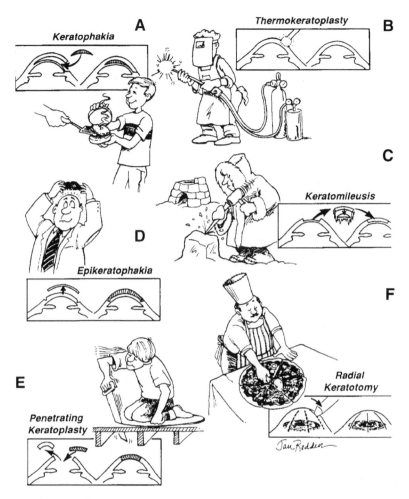

Figure 8–1 Some of the principal procedures for refractive corneal surgery shown allegorically.
    (A) Keratophakia: Similar to filling a roast beef sandwich.
    (B) Thermokeratoplasty: Similar to welding a metallic seam.
    (C) Keratomileusis: Similar to trimming an ice block.
    (D) Epikeratophakia: Similar to patching a bald spot.
    (E) Penetrating keratoplasty: Similar to transplanting a shrub graft.
    (F) Radial keratotomy: Similar to an eight-segment pizza cutting.

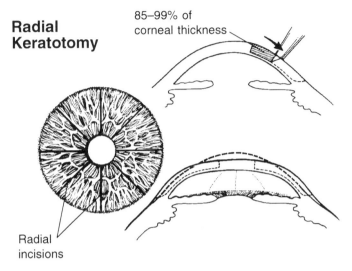

Radial Keratotomy

Radial incisions

85–99% of corneal thickness

Figure 8–2 Note the radial incisions made so as to leave a completely unincised clear central zone. Incisions are cut up to 90 percent through the stroma.

better. These temporary problems can be treated with one or more special glasses or contacts, as needed. They are a small price to pay for the improved sight achieved.

Middle-aged people commonly discover that their eyes' capacity to focus on close objects has diminished by the phenomenon known as *presbyopia*. Those who were already myopic will not be affected as much with this change in vision since they frequently take their glasses off to read and eat.

Since surgery can't do much about tissue changes, an operation to correct focal length problems must hone in on what the individual wants to see with the exposed eye. Most people prefer to have the correction made for ordinary activities, such as walking the dog or driving to work. For moderate to very close seeing, as for reading or model building, half-glasses or bifocals in full glasses may be needed. For those who are nearsighted but use their eyes at close range most of the day, such as draftsmen, machinists, and secretaries, you may decide not to have surgery and simply continue wearing glasses for ordinary activities like watching a large-screen movie or driving to and from work.

Odd as it may seem at first thought, some individuals opt to have one eye corrected for distance while the other is left for close work. In this way, the balance of binocular vision is corrected for far or near with single refractive glasses or contacts. This type of correction is referred to as *monovision.* Prior to surgery it is wise to attempt wearing a contact lens in only one eye to experience this near/far correction. Those who find that they cannot tolerate a monovision contact lens correction after a pre-op trial period of a few days must decide whether or not to pass on an operation altogether or have both eyes surgically corrected.

Your age has a lot to do with how predictably healing will occur after RK. Since healing is not as fast or complete with increasing age, surgeons are inclined to use fewer incisions for a grandfather than for a middle-aged man. Even more incisions are needed for his 20-year-old grandson. Even by age 50, the rates of bodily decline are variable enough for individual health characteristics to make a difference in what a surgeon will decide to attempt.

There are also individual characteristics unique to heredity, which influence how appropriate RK may be. If the thickness of the cornea is shallow, as measured by *pachymetry,* there may not be enough depth of tissue to work with. Also, the cornea may be abnormally steep and conical, or *keratoconic.* The surgeon may study computer-produced charts to help in a diagnosis of this condition. If it is extreme, a keratoconic cornea is so stretched and thinned here and there that RK will usually not produce satisfactory results.

Intraocular pressure (IOP) is another variable influencing the success of RK. A high IOP is generally associated with overcorrection and/or progressive farsightedness in RK patients. Low IOP, on the other hand, produces the same effect in the eye as an under-inflated tire or balloon with less "pooching outward." The effects of RK can be diminished by the decreased IOP. As the incision scars heal and produce excessive contraction, the results of the operation are reversed. For whatever it is worth in our time of fairly common illegal drug use, marijuana is known to produce low IOP in the course of offering the user an "out of focus" world. For those who are users despite all warnings, don't smoke for three months prior to surgery or for a year afterward if you want a shot at successful RK. Here's a positive thought: the time abstaining may help you kick the habit and get into something better like low-stress aerobics.

Perhaps the most important single contraindication to refractive surgery is your mental frame of mind and your expectations. This surgery is not an exact science. There is no iron-clad guarantee of surgery leading to 20/20 vision without glasses (emmetropia). Your ophthalmologist will do his or her best in pre-op examinations and planning to make you happy with your vision. The ophthalmologist will be careful not to "overshoot," leading to excessive farsightedness (hyperopia). The optimum is to correct you to just shy of 20/20 vision, leaving just a touch of myopia with vision good enough so that glasses or contact lenses are not needed for driving. If only perfect 20/20 vision is acceptable to you, then surgery should not be performed. Remember that the primary goal is to "improve organ function."

The RK procedure has greatly improved regarding safety and predictability with the advent of new ultra-thin diamond knives (see Fig. 8–3), computer programs, and a vast base of experience.

The success rate of RK (1994) is very high in the low to moderate refractive correction range of –1.00 to –6.00 diopters. A suitable patient has about a 90–95 percent chance of being able to obtain an unrestricted driver's license (20/40 or better). High degrees of nearsightedness (approximately –7.00 or –8.00 or greater) are generally beyond the capability of the procedure although exceptional situations do exist. RK is an outpatient procedure done under local anesthesia which, when combined with topical (Ocufen™, Acular™, Voltaren™) and oral nonsteroidal anti-inflammatory drugs (Motrin™, Voltaren™, Ansaid™), causes almost no pain. Patients are generally able to return to work in about two to three days.

Statistically, about three percent of patients will be disappointed with the RK results. Disappointment comes from overcorrection (hyperopia), undercorrection (still slightly nearsighted) and induced astigmatism (caused from the surgery). "Starburst," "halo," and

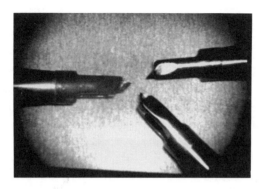

Figure 8–3   Example of diamond knives used for radial keratotomy.

"glare" effects, and "fluctuations" in vision are also troublesome, although temporary. Overcorrections cannot be treated well at this writing, but a number of techniques including excimer laser, holmium laser, and automated lamellar keratectomy or keratoplasty (ALK) are currently developing programs for these situations. A more conservative approach termed "titratable" RK is now taught and is being performed by some surgeons. In this approach, only four incisions are made in each stage of the surgery. This technique may be helpful in preventing overcorrections. The disadvantage is that you may need up to four or five procedures per eye to achieve the desired corrections. These procedures are done incrementally over a period of time.

Undercorrections and/or astigmatism can usually be improved by doing one or more "adjustment" or "enhancement" procedures later. The chance of needing such a procedure is about 10 percent using standard non-titratable techniques.

Success factors for individual patients can be partially determined from the corneal curvature, or "K's," and present glasses prescription. The cornea can generally be flattened to a 38.00 diopter curve in RK. If your K's are 44.00 and the contact lens prescription is a –4.50 diopters, there exists a good chance for full correction. In explanation, 44.00 minus 4.50 leaves a post-operative cornea of 39.50, which is steeper than the flatter 38.00. Surgery in this instance should be successful. Significant undercorrections may be fixed in the future with excimer or ALK procedures.

In all candor, there are possible complications from RK (in addition to simple infections) which need to be acknowledged. In spite of all care, the normal incisions which go 95 percent of the distance through the cornea may inadvertently prick through it and cause an increased chance of an *endophthalmitis* infection. The other problem is *progressive hyperopia.* If the cornea fails to heal as predicted, it can stretch too far and become excessively flat, making the eye farsighted. This has been the case for about one in 200 patients, and is possibly closely related to those who develop glaucoma. A careful review of glaucoma in the family and its discussion with your surgeon is indicated. It sounds worse than it is, for these patients usually do fine wearing a contact lens on the eye in question.

Vision after RK may vary during the day. Usually the variance is small. In rare cases, the vision may fluctuate so severely after RK surgery that two or three sets of glasses or contacts are needed. This is caused by fluid entering the cornea and producing swelling. Thus, the corneal shape and power is changed. Areas of the epithelium which are not tightly adherent to your cornea, and hence are not waterproof, are the usual cause of these severe fluctuations. These abnormal areas of loose epithelium are called *recurrent epithelial erosions.* These defects in the waterproof layer allow tears to penetrate inside the cornea from the outside.

If one of the incisions is too deep, the aqueous from inside the eye can enter the corneal stroma, causing localized corneal edema. This edema is a common culprit that produces visual fluctuations. Ointment at bedtime or a continuous-wear bandage soft contact lens generally stabilizes the eye and facilitates healing. If a continuous-wear soft contact lens does not stabilize the perforated endothelium, a simple suture may be required to remedy the problem. Statistically, radial keratotomy has proved to be an excellent procedure.

Excimer Laser

This is a relatively new procedure in which focused pulses of "cold laser" light called photons are projected onto the front surface of the cornea while the patient looks at a target. The strongly energized photons cut material by breaking the weak carbon-carbon bonds in the cornea, like a molecular knife. Computerized programs, shutters, and masks are being developed to produce a variety of shapes to correct most refractive errors. The exact roles and magnitude of correction have not yet been determined. The advantages of this technique are many. The "incision" or "sculpting" is only 10 percent or less of the corneal thickness compared to much deeper cutting in other techniques. Your corneal stroma ablates at a known rate, allowing a computer calculated treatment to be designed. The machine is a computer-controlled "robolaser" requiring much less surgical skill and experience than RK, ALK, or other procedures. Surgical laser times are short, only 10 to 40 seconds with the patient actually in the room about 15 minutes. Initial results are very good. Our patients, three years after surgery, have been stable, and 93 percent see 20/20 or better, with most of them seeing one or two lines better than 20/20. No progressive hyperopia occurs with this technique. Some concern exists about possible long-term corneal haze and refractive stability. After five years, the eyes see well and look well. The cost is fairly high, however; the laser costs over $400,000 with maintenance costs of over $50,000 per year as these words are written.

Refractive Lamellar Keratoplasties

The first group of procedures have been given the name *partial thickness keratoplasty*. The latter word comes from the Greek "kerato" referring to the cornea and "plasty" implying remolding or reshaping. "Partial" signifies that the surgery is only partway through the cornea in contrast to a *penetrating keratoplasty* which goes all the way through the cornea (see Fig. 8–1E).

Another term used for the first sub-area of corneal refractive surgery is *lamellar keratoplasty*. The word *lamellar* comes from the Latin "lamella" meaning leaf. This type of surgery involves using carefully shaped thin layers of the cornea called *lenticules* to position inside or use as covers for the patient's cornea (see Fig. 8–1A).

There are a number of refractive procedures that are forms of *lamellar keratoplasty*. These types of surgeries involve utilizing carefully shaped, thin layers of cornea called "lenticules" to position inside your cornea or use as refractive covers for the patient's cornea. These are used to solve refractive problems felt to be of moderate or high proportions, generally minus five diopters or greater.

Keratomileusis

The initial corneal lathing procedure, *myopic keratomileusis* (MKM) was developed in the late 1950s by Jose Barroquer, M.D., and later Luis Ruiz, M.D., in Bogota, Colombia (Fig. 8–4 and Fig. 8–1C).

In MKM a special high-speed corneal lathe removes a top "button" or "disc" of approximately 50 percent of the corneal thickness. The button is then placed on a special lathe, frozen and ground like a contact lens, reshaping the corneal disc to yield the necessary and precise refractive power. After thawing, the corneal button with the "new power" is replaced on the eye and sutured in place. This technique is extremely difficult, but well-done procedures produce excellent results with almost no pain or discomfort. Vision is usually excellent in one to seven days. Problems with irregular astigmatism and cells in the graft interface (the junction between the cap and the eye) are sometimes associated with the procedure.

In another type of lamellar keratoplasty called *epikeratophakia,* the outermost layer of the patient's cornea, the epithelium, is scraped off and a fresh or frozen lenticule from a human donor's cornea is shaped to the desired refractive specifications and grafted on top of the scraped cornea of the patient. It is similar to putting a tire patch over a bald spot on an auto tire (see Fig. 8–1D).

Automated Lamellar Keratoplasty

This is a new and simpler version of MKM. In ALK, instead of freezing and lathing the corneal button, a second lathing across the cornea corrects your error. The cap or button is then repositioned back into place and generally sutures are not needed. Computer programs calculate the exact amount of lathing required to produce the new refraction. When the cap or button is repositioned onto the cornea, the total thickness of the cornea in the center is less, making

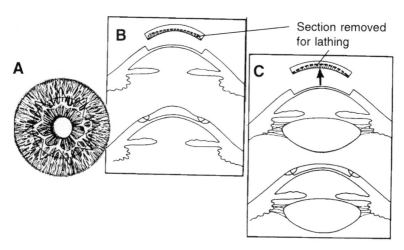

Figure 8–4   Keratomileusis procedure shown for nearsighted and farsighted eyes.
(A) Front view of the eye after a keratomileusis procedure.
(B) Keratomileusis for a hyperopic eye after the lens has been removed (aphakic eye). The cornea is thicker centrally, reducing farsightedness.
(C) Keratomileusis for a myopic eye. The cornea is thinner centrally, reducing nearsightedness.

the front curve flatter, or the eye less nearsighted. Vision is restored within several days, and sometimes restored the next day. There is essentially no discomfort.

This simpler procedure was begun on a large scale in early 1993. No long-term statistics are yet available. Problems resulting from this procedure have been the loss of the button and epithelial cells, or cysts accidentally implanted in between the button and the cut surface of the eye (the "interface"). Irregular astigmatism is also another problem. Exact power predictions have not yet been possible, hence many patients need a follow up RK to adjust residual nearsightedness and/or astigmatism. A variation of ALK currently being studied involves using the excimer laser to produce the correction in the stroma while the cap is off. The cap is then repositioned onto the freshly lasered cornea and no sutures are necessary. Initial results look very good and vision is excellent within one to several days.

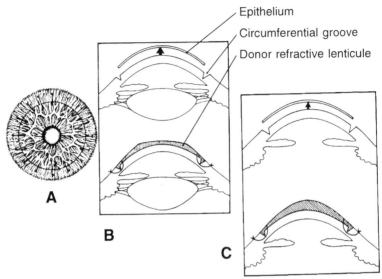

Figure 8–5   Epikeratophakia procedure shown for nearsighted and farsighted eyes.
(A) Front view of the eye after an epikeratophakia procedure.
(B) Epikeratophiakia for a myopic eye. The donor lenticule is thinner centrally, decreasing myopia (nearsightedness).
(C) Epikeratophakia for a hyperopic eye in a patient who is also aphakic (having no lens as in previous cataract extraction without IOL). The donor lenticule is thicker centrally, decreasing hyperopia (farsightedness).

Epikeratophakia

In other types of lamellar procedures, the outermost layer of your cornea, the epithelium, is scraped and removed (see Fig. 8–5). In this procedure, a frozen, dehydrated, or a fresh lenticule from a human donor is shaped to the desired refractive specifications and grafted on top of your cornea. A small groove area in the edge of your cornea allows the edges of the graft to be "tucked in" and the corneal graft to be sutured in place for healing. John Goosey, M.D., in Houston is currently doing an FDA study, which includes chil-

Corneal Refractive Surgery

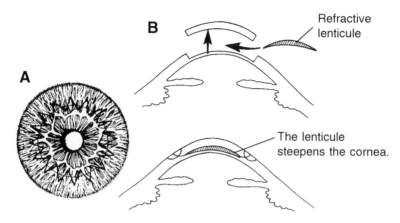

Figure 8–6   Keratophakia procedure for a hyperopic eye.
(A) Front view of the eye after a keratophakia procedure.
(B) The lenticule is thicker centrally, thus increasing the corneal power. Keratophakia is the equivalent of adding plus eyeglasses or contact lenses in the visual axis.

dren, because they are not good candidates for refractive surgery or intraocular lens implants, referred to as *keratomileusis in situ*, using fresh corneas. This procedure seems to work in keratoconus, a condition where the cornea begins thinning and stretching out of shape.

In yet another type of lamellar keratoplasty, called *keratophakia*, a lenticule from a human donor or a synthetically made lenticule is placed inside the recipient's cornea. This can be done by removing a corneal cap and inserting the lenticule underneath the cap which is then sutured back into place. In the other technique, a special corneal pocket in the cornea is created to contain the lenticule and the edge of the pocket is then sutured. Please see Fig. 8–6 above and Fig. 8–1A on page 115.

Refractive Corneal Keratectomy

Another older refractive procedure uses the suffix "ectomy" as in appendectomy. "Ectomy" means cutting and removal. In this case, an incision is made near the limbus and a thin sliver of cornea is excised. The wound is carefully sutured together causing the flat curve of cornea to become much steeper. This is a powerful technique and it is useful in cases of severe astigmatism.

Penetrating Corneal Keratoplasty (Corneal Transplant)

Penetrating corneal keratoplasty as compared to partial thickness keratoplasty is used when describing corneal transplants. In this procedure, the whole cornea is excised and removed. It is then replaced by a healthy human donor cornea. This must be done when the vital endothelial cell layer has been badly damaged or when corneal scar tissue, haze, or surface irregularities have developed to the point that you cannot see through your cornea. A further discussion follows in the Corneal and External Disease chapter (Chapter Eleven).

Thermal Keratoplasty/Holmium Laser Thermal Keratotomy

In these procedures, a heat source is utilized to correct corneal refractive irregularities by spot heat-treatment commonly referred to as *thermokeratoplasty* (Fig.8–1B, page 115). The heat is used to shrink or contract the corneal stromal collagen fibers which serve as the chief structural component of the main layer of the cornea. The contraction of the fibers around the periphery of the cornea steepens the cornea, thus altering its shape and power. The first units and procedures were done by Dr. Fyodorov in about 1985. Their reported results were good but they have been unable as yet to secure FDA approval for their machine in the U.S.A. A hand-held holmium laser tip, which is carefully positioned in predetermined patterns on the cornea, promises to be a more sophisticated, reliable, and reproducible modification of Dr. Fyodorov's concept. The computer/laser interaction is able to measure and calculate the thermal heating more accurately than the Russian device. Currently, FDA

Corneal Refractive Surgery

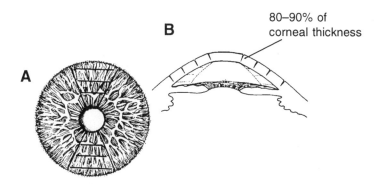

Figure 8–7   Ruiz procedure to correct or reduce astigmatism.
(A) Front view of the eye following a Ruiz procedure.
(B) Pattern of incisions used for a Ruiz trapezoidal keratotomy for severe astigmatism, flattened at 12 and 6 o'clock.

investigations of this procedure at Summit Technology, Inc., are underway in the United States.

Hyperopic Hexagonal Keratotomy

This is a procedure where six "pinwheel" incisions around the optical axis are performed by cutting the stromal fibers loose. The central fibers contract and steepen the central button. This makes the central corneal curve steeper and, therefore, more powerful. The focal point of light is consequently moved forward in the eye. Remember, a hyperope's eyes are "too short." While this procedure is conceptually clear, it is difficult to perform and is not reproducible. There are only a few highly skilled surgeons who can successfully perform this procedure.

Ruiz Procedure

This special trapezoidal pattern or ladder-shaped procedure can correct up to six diopters of astigmatism. This is a special RK pattern (Fig. 8–7).

Wrap-Up

- Refractive surgery is defined as a surgical procedure which alters how the eye focuses light onto the retina. It is meant to decrease or eliminate your dependence on corrective lenses, such as eyeglasses or contact lenses.
- More than 95 percent of patients seeking refractive surgery have the procedure done for personal safety and functional reasons not cosmetic reasons.
- Cataract surgery is the most common refractive surgery performed today. Radial keratotomy (RK) is the second most frequent.
- Ninety-seven percent of radial keratotomy patients are significantly improved and happy with their surgery results.
- Starburst, halo, glare, and fluctuations in corneal power are all associated with RK. Fortunately, most of these visual disturbances diminish in two weeks and are completely gone in approximately four months.
- If you are presbyopic, or soon will be, additional time and explanation may be spent with you, since there are several visual considerations of which you need to be aware.
- Some patients in their late 30s and 40s who are considering refractive surgery may wish to simulate presbyopia after surgery by wearing a contact lens on one or both eyes.
- Excimer laser is currently under FDA study and initial results are excellent.
- Automated lamellar keratectomy (ALK) is an effective, almost painless procedure capable of correcting up to 20 plus diopters of nearsightedness, and two to five diopters of farsightedness. Long-term results and statistical success are still unknown, but initial results are excellent.

Chapter Nine

Diseases and Surgery of the Retina

Keith A. Bourgeois

Physiology of Sight

The retina can be likened to film in a camera. Light travels first through the transparent cornea, second to the aperture created by the iris, and finally through the lens and the vitreous. At the end of this journey, it reaches the retinal surface, where electrochemical processes change the light into impulses, which travel along the optic nerve to the brain. The impulses ultimately end up in the part of the brain called the *occipital visual cortex*. This cortex is underneath the occipital bone of the skull, which you can find with your finger. It is the large bump behind the ear. It is here where the impulses are actually processed into what we know as sight.

The retina extends from the border of the optic nerve to a few millimeters behind the iris. The front of the retina, which is closest to the iris, is called the peripheral retina and is important because it is relatively thin and may develop holes or tears. The portion of the retina that is furthest from the front of the eye is called the *macula*. There is a small zone in the direct center of the macula called the *fovea*. The fovea is unique because it contains no retinal blood vessels. The macula is responsible for our 20/20 vision and is important because the macula is where the center of an object is focused on the retina. For example, if you are looking at someone's face, the center of the face is focused on the macula. This is important to understand because there are disorders of the central retina, or macula, that rob people of central vision and fine visual acuity. If your retina is not diseased outside of the macula, you would maintain peripheral vision. Vision with only the peripheral retina is usually about 20/200.

Age-Related Macular Degeneration

The most common disorder of the macula is called *age-related macular degeneration* (ARMD), or in less politically correct former times called senile macular degeneration. In this case senile meant occurring in older adults. It did not imply any change in mental capacity. The word "degeneration" signifies a progressive deterioration leading to decreased function in an organ or tissue. The area of the retina affected in ARMD is usually limited to the macula. There are two main forms of age-related macular degeneration commonly called *dry* and *wet*. In the more common dry form, the diagnosis is based on the appearance of the macula during an eye exam. The doctor sees small yellow flecks in the macula that are called drusen (Fig. 9–1). There are also pale or dark spots caused by a clumping or thinning of the pigmented layer of the retina. Although smaller, these spots are similar to age spots on the skin. A retina that demonstrates these degenerative changes is actually thinner, and termed *atrophic*. Through these areas of the atrophic retina, there occasionally grows an abnormal network of blood vessels from the underlining layer called the *choroid*. The choroid is an important layer of blood vessels located between the retina and the sclera, which is the tough, fibrous, white outer coat of the eye. Along with the choroid's other duties, it functions as a transporter of nutrients and carrier of waste from the retina. When the blood vessels from the choroid grow into the retina, they cause scarring that leads to permanent visual loss. This ingrowth of blood vessels from the choroid is called a *choroidal neovascular membrane*

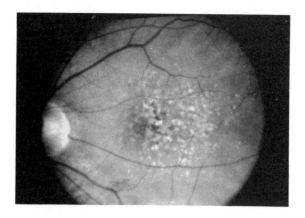

Figure 9–1 This photograph exhibits the dry form of age-related macular degeneration with drusen.

(CNVM) (Fig. 9–2). When this scenario occurs, it converts dry into wet-age related macular degeneration. A dye called fluorescein is injected into a vein, usually in the arm, in order to take photos of the intraocular circulation in the macular region to aid in locating choroidal neovascular membranes. This procedure is called a *fluorescein angiogram* and is usually performed in a doctor's office. Approximately one or two out of 10 of the patients that have the dry form of age-related macular degeneration will have the misfortune to develop a choroidal neovascular membrane. If the choroidal neovascular membrane occurs in one eye there is a much higher risk of it developing in the other eye. In developed countries, age-related macular degeneration is the most common cause of legal blindness in people over 60 years of age. Most legal blindness is caused by the wet form of age-related macular degeneration. Central vision may be severely diminished even in the dry form of this condition because of extensive atrophy, but typically in dry age-related macular degeneration, the patient can still read about half of the letters on an eye chart.

It is important to realize that patients suffering from macular degeneration are not completely blind. The central vision is missing or severely distorted, but the peripheral vision remains. This explains

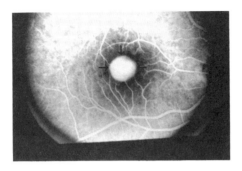

Figure 9–2 Fluorescein angiography photograph showing a severe choroidal neovascular membrane.

why people with ARMD can't read or recognize faces but can navigate successfully around all the furniture in a room. With ARMD it is actually harder to see nearer objects than those far away.

There is presently no known treatment for the dry form of macular degeneration. Currently, there is research under way to determine if the rate of deterioration seen in ARMD may be delayed by taking vitamins and minerals by mouth. Vitamins and minerals, such as vitamins A and E, are known to be important for normal retinal functioning, but it is not known if taking extra vitamins will have a beneficial visual effect on the sick retina in ARMD.

The only currently available non-experimental treatment for wet ARMD is *laser photocoagulation* (Fig. 9–3). The laser most commonly used is the argon, which coagulates the new blood vessels along with the overlying retina. A small surrounding area of normal retina is also destroyed to lessen the chance of recurrence. Unfortunately, when the choroidal neovascular membrane is beneath the fovea, laser treatment is likely to make the vision worse. The benefit of laser treatment is a reduction of the size of the blind spot when compared over time to individuals with a CNVM who have not had laser treatment. A greater visual benefit is seen in eyes lucky enough to have the choroidal neovascular membrane far away from the center of the macula. The closer the membrane occurs to the center of the macula, which is called the fovea, the worse the visual outcome, either with or without laser treatment. A common occur-

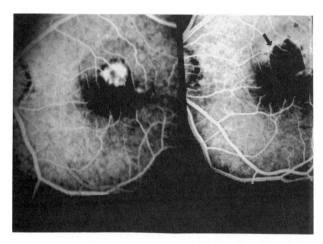

Figure 9-3 The fluorescein angiography photograph on the left shows wet ARMD, where the black area is a hemorrhage, and the white area is a CNVM. The fluorescein angiography photograph on the right (arrow) shows the CNVM after it has been obliterated by laser treatment.

rence, which is a tremendous disappointment, is the regrowth of the choroidal neovascular membrane. Weeks or months after a successful laser treatment, this growth may occur in another area of the retina or may occur adjacent to the area of previous laser treatment. The recurrence of the choroidal neovascular membrane develops in 60 percent of eyes within two years after successful destruction of the first membrane with laser treatment. Due to this high recurrence rate with laser therapy, many experimental treatments are currently being investigated including medicines, surgery, and even radiation therapy.

There are other conditions that can develop choroidal neovascularization and can cause a similar visual loss as seen in wet ARMD. Common causes include trauma, parasitic infections, such as *histoplasmosis* and *toxoplasmosis* (Fig. 9-4) or even extreme nearsightedness (myopia). In traumatic injuries, cracks may develop in the deep layers of the retina. This type of injury is called a *choroidal rupture* and may develop CNVM. Histoplasmosis is a

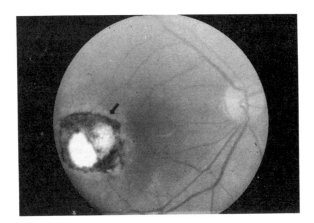

Figure 9–4   Toxoplasmosis in the macular area.

parasitic retinal infection that occurs in the United States, most commonly in the Ohio and Mississippi River basins. These scars may develop a CNVM. Very nearsighted people have extremely long eyeballs. In this high myopia, cracks may develop in the retina from the stress of progressive elongation of the eye as the person gets more nearsighted. These are called *lacquer cracks* because of the similarity of cracks in the finish of antique furniture. Occasionally, even the back of the sclera gets so thin from this stretching that an outward bulge forms which is called a *staphyloma*. The staphyloma and resulting lacquer cracks are called *myopic degeneration*. All of these disorders share the common feature of an area of damage in the retina that can allow for ingrowth of blood vessels from the underlying choroid. If a CNVM occurs in this damaged area, a scar may develop very similar to wet macular degeneration and cause a blind spot.

Diabetic Retinopathy

After having diabetes for a few years, most people develop damage to small blood vessels in many places throughout the body. Examples of this include tingling in the hands and feet, decreased kidney function, cardiovascular and cerebrovascular problems, and changes in the retina called *diabetic retinopathy*. Diabetic retinopathy is divided into background and proliferative types.

Background diabetic retinopathy is more common and is seen in 90 percent of people who have had diabetes for approximately 20 years. Background diabetic retinopathy is characterized by the formation of small sack-like outgrowths of the retinal capillaries called *microaneurysms*. When viewed by your doctor these sacks look like a round red dot and under a microscope resemble an egg forming on a tire innertube. These can burst, causing small retinal hemorrhages, and may form clots leading to a lack of blood flow in the retina. Because of the thinness of the walls in a microaneurysm, there can be a leakage of the fluid called serum or plasma into the retina. *Retinal edema* occurs when these vessels leak. In pumping this fluid out of the retina, small yellow clumps of protein and fat are left behind, which are called *hard exudates*. The central area of the retina is often where this type of leakage occurs causing decreased central vision. Laser treatment called *focal macular photocoagulation* can diminish the rate of visual loss by reducing this macular edema. Laser surgery, which cauterizes the leaking microaneurysms, usually is performed after topical anesthetic eyedrops have been instilled.

Because of poor circulation in the retina from diabetes, some people grow abnormal new blood vessels on the retinal surface that are called *retinal neovascularization*. When this serious condition occurs, it converts background to *proliferative diabetic retinopathy*. *Retinal neovascularization* vessels are more fragile than normal blood vessels and tend to bleed, causing clumps of blood in a normally clear vitreous gel. These clumps may clear with the passage of time. Retinal neovascularization vessels also tend to grow in clumps that band together, forming fibrous strands that can cause severe loss of sight from retinal detachment. Luckily, there are treatments that can cause regression of this retinal neovascularization and thus reduce the rate of vision loss. A type of laser treatment called *pan retinal photocoagulation* (PRP) is used if there is a clear enough view through the blood and vitreous (Fig. 9–5). This is an outpatient laser surgery performed in the office or hospital outpatient laser

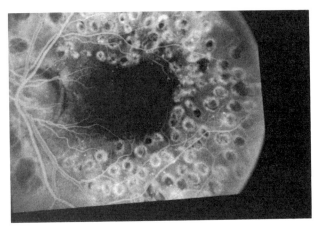

Figure 9–5 Shows the retinal appearance after it has been treated with pan-retinal photocoagulation for proliferative diabetic retinopathy.

room. PRP is performed either with topical anesthesia using eye drops or local anesthetic injection.

If there is non-clearing vitreous hemorrhage or a retinal detachment has occurred in proliferative diabetic retinopathy, then a surgery called *vitrectomy* is recommended. In a vitrectomy, small, delicate instruments are inserted into the eye that remove the blood and fibrous scars. After the blood is removed and the retina reattached, a small fiberoptic tube from a laser is inserted into the eye to perform the same pattern of photocoagulation as seen in pan retinal photocoagulation. This laser is called *endophotocoagulation* and is performed in the operating room. Vitrectomy and endophotocoagulation may either be performed under general anesthesia or local injection.

Additional Macular Problems

There are other diseases that affect the macula and cause decreased central vision. A round hole can form in the central macula. These holes are called *macular holes* and are usually present in only one eye in the affected patient. The risk of developing a macular hole in the fellow eye is about 10 percent. A macular hole causes a blind spot with a sharp border in the central vision. The image formed is like a puzzle missing some pieces in the center. The cause of these holes is believed to be the traction of the retina by the vitreous. Recently, we have learned that the blind spot may enlarge over time because of a small surrounding retinal detachment caused by this hole. A vitrectomy surgery along with instillation of intraocular gas may recover some vision. This surgery can decrease the size of the blind spot and regain some visual acuity in 60 percent of patients. The patient must maintain face-down positioning for two weeks following the surgery. The purpose of the inactivity is to help position the gas bubble over the hole to aid in healing.

Another condition that affects the macula is a thin, shiny-surfaced, opaque membrane that grows over the macula and causes distortion of the normally smooth surface. This condition is usually called a *macular pucker* in order to describe the surface wrinkling caused by this membrane. Another name used to describe this condition is *cellophane retinopathy* because of the shiny surface. There is a surgery called *vitrectomy* and *membrane peeling* which may reclaim some vision. In this surgery, intraocular forceps, which are like small pliers, are used to peel the membrane off the retinal surface. Complications from this surgery include bleeding and tears in the retina. Occasionally, these complications cause a post-operative loss in visual acuity.

Age-related degeneration, macular holes, and macular pucker occur most commonly in older adults. *Central serous retinopathy* (also known as "central serous choroidopathy") is a macular disorder that is most commonly seen in young adults (Fig. 9–6). A blister of fluid containing serum develops in the macula, causing a central visual distortion. Most describe this distortion as if there is a water drop on the central part of their glasses. Fortunately, most of these blisters will dry out over several months with complete or virtually complete restoration of vision. A laser treatment has been shown to hasten the resolution of this condition by a few weeks, but does not have any effect on the eventual visual outcome. In central serous retinopathy, a fluorescein angiogram might be used to show where

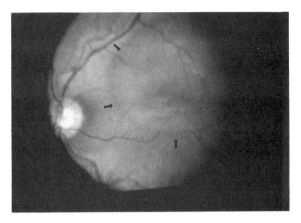

Figure 9–6   Large central serous retinopathy (inside arrows).

the abnormal leakage is located. Approximately 40 percent of eyes with one episode of central serous retinopathy will get central serous retinopathy again in the same eye at some time in the future. Forty percent will also contract central serous retinopathy in the other previously non-affected eye at some time in the future.

Retinal Detachment

A devastating cause of visual loss is retinal detachment. Most detachments of the retina occur when a small hole or tear develops in the peripheral retina. Why such a break develops in the retina is unknown. Sometimes these breaks are caused by blunt trauma such as being hit in the eye with a ball or a fist. In other detachments, these retinal breaks arise spontaneously without any precipitating cause. Another condition that may occasionally develop into a retinal detachment is called *lattice degeneration*. Lattice degeneration is named for areas of thinning in the peripheral retina. These areas are present in approximately five percent of the population and are more common in myopic (nearsighted) people. These areas tend to develop retinal holes more easily than normal eyes. Symptoms of retinal detachment include flashes of light, floaters, and a veil-like vision loss. There is no pain. Fluid from the vitreous flows through the break in the retina and causes separation in the retinal layers. If caught in an early stage, a laser or a freezing probe can be used to make a scar around the retinal break that will act as a barrier to further detachment. This type of treatment is usually performed with topical eyedrops or a local anesthetic injection under the conjunctiva. When performed with a laser it is referred to as *laser retinopexy*, and when performed with the freezing probe it is referred to as *cryopexy*.

When a detachment is too large, the most common type of surgery used to repair the retina is a *scleral buckle*. In this surgery, a plastic band is sutured to the sclera. The fluid between the sclera and the retina may be drained. The band is tightened, producing an indentation or "buckling" of the sclera sufficient to re-establish contact with the separated retina. Once the retina and sclera are touching, the scleral buckle acts as a bolster to allow for laser or freezing treatments to form beneficial adhesions between the previously separated retinal layers. These adhesions close the flow of fluid through the retinal break. A scleral buckle is performed under general or local anesthesia. An alternative treatment for retinal detachment is *pneumatic retinopexy*. Pneumatic retinopexy utilizes an expanding gas bubble as an internal bolster which presses the retina outward against the sclera. The retinal break is then closed with the aid of laser or freezing therapy. Both of the above treatments are equally successful in causing retinal reattachment in approximately 85 percent of patients. Your surgeon will explain why one of these may be more beneficial to you based upon the characteristics of your retinal detachment. The amount of visual recovery depends upon the duration of the detachment and what areas of the retina are involved. Since a detachment may enlarge quickly, it is important to visit your eye doctor promptly when visual problems are first noticed.

Another form of retinal detachment is a *tractional retinal detachment*. In this type of retinal detachment, there is not a tear or hole in the retina. The detachment occurs from strands that form in the vitreous and pull on the retina. These strands in the vitreous sometimes form in response to a retinal detachment and can occasionally get worse after uncomplicated retinal detachment surgery. The strands in the vitreous are similar to adhesions that may form in the abdomen in response to hemorrhage or inflammation from diseases. When this type of scar occurs in the eye it is called *proliferative vitreo-retinopathy* (PVR). Proliferative vitreo-retinopathy is the leading cause of retinal surgery failure. About one-half of the eyes that fail initial surgical repair of the retina can be successfully reattached with repeated surgery. Surgical procedures for complex retinal detachments usually include vitrectomy, endophotocoagulation, and an intraocular gas bubble. It is not uncommon to require multiple surgeries in order to treat proliferative vitreo-retinopathy. Vitrectomy means surgical removal of the vitreous. In this case, care is taken to excise all vitreous strands that are causing traction on the retina. The main reason for the retina to often detach again in this type of surgery is that the strands may grow back. Laser treatments and different types of intraocular gas bubbles are used to increase the chance of retinal repair. The surgeon has a variety of gases which last different intervals inside the eye. Some gases last from a few days to over a month. All gases are absorbed by the eye, and surgery is not needed to remove them.

In severe cases of retinal detachment, a non-absorbing bubble containing silicone oil is used instead of an absorbable gas bubble. This has the advantage of providing a long-acting support for the retina, but it has the disadvantage of requiring surgical removal when the retina is sufficiently healed.

HIV and the Retina

Recently, severe vision problems are occurring due to an eye infection developing in patients infected with the HIV virus, which causes *Acquired Immune Deficiency Syndrome* (AIDS). This condition is referred to as *cytomegalovirus* (CMV) retinitis. CMV is an infection of the retina that can be slowed by utilizing intravenous medication, but not eradicated. The retinal infection can eat through the retina in places, causing retinal detachment from multiple small holes. Repair of this unusual detachment is usually with vitrectomy and silicone oil.

Retinitis pigmentosa is an inherited disease that causes progressive visual loss. It is named pigmentosa because clumps of pigment are

Diseases and Surgery of the Retina

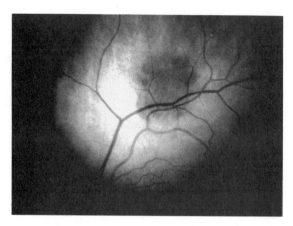

Figure 9–7 A harmless choroidal nevus which has developed in the retina.

seen in the retina during an eye exam. Typically, adults develop increasingly narrow visual fields that resemble looking through a gun barrel. This often progresses to legal blindness. A recent study revealed that adult patients may slow the rate of their visual loss by taking oral vitamin A.

A condition that mimics symptoms of retinal detachment is a *posterior vitreous detachment*, or PVD. In a PVD, the vitreous gel pulls forward off the optic nerve and posterior retina. This causes floaters and rarely may cause tears in the retina. There is no treatment available for the floaters, but they usually diminish over time.

Various pigmented lesions occur in the retina. The most common is called a *choroidal nevus* and is similar to a mole on the skin (Fig. 9–7). Just like moles of the skin, there is a slight chance that a choroidal nevus might undergo a malignant change. The cancer that may arise from a benign choroidal nevus is a malignant melanoma. The treatment for malignant melanoma of the eye formerly included surgical removal of the eye. This surgical removal of the eye is called an *enucleation*. Currently, investigation is in progress on a surgery delivering radiation therapy, as well as other therapies which may encourage regression of this tumor, thereby avoiding loss of the eye in some cases.

Wrap-Up

- The macula is the area in the back of the eye which allows you to see fine detail and color vision.
- The fovea is the center of the macula responsible for our 20/20 vision.
- Age-related macular degeneration (ARMD) is the most common disorder of the macula.
- ARMD has two basic forms, commonly called "wet" or "dry."
- Ninety to 95 percent of individuals having ARMD are of the "dry" type and no significant treatment other than low vision aids are possible. Antioxidants, such as Vitamins C and E, and selenium may be of minimal, if any, help.
- Wet ARMD can sometimes be treated with lasers. Unfortunately, the long-term visual prognosis is poor.
- As a group, diabetes is the most common endocrine disorder. Diabetes is also the leading cause of new blindness in the United States.
- In diabetes mellitus, abnormal new blood vessels, which are thin-walled and frail, may develop in the retina, causing diabetic retinopathy. These new blood vessels may leak fluid or hemorrhage into your eye, causing decreased vision.
- Most diabetic retinopathy begins 11 to 20 years after insulin treatment begins.
- Pan retinal laser photocoagulation is effective in managing proliferative diabetic retinopathy. In severe cases, vitrectomy and laser photocoagulation may be necessary.
- If you develop retinal problems due to poor blood circulation, one baby aspirin taken every other day (if not medically contraindicated) may significantly decrease your chances of visual problems.
- Signs and symptoms of retinal detachment are painless and may include a sudden onset of flashes of light, black floaters, and/or a "veil" or "curtain" across your vision.

- Scleral buckling procedures are used to repair significant retinal detachments and are successful in 85 percent of the cases.
- Histoplasmosis is a highly infectious fungus that usually causes an acute non-fatal benign infection, but which can infect the eyes in childhood. As adults, a subretinal neovascular membrane may develop in the scars.
- Choroidal melanoma is eight times more common in Caucasians than in African-Americans and three times more common in Asian populations.

Chapter Ten

Pediatric Eye Care

Lawrence Lynn and Warren D. Cross

Disorders in Newborns

The treatment of children's eyes poses special difficulties, especially for pre-schoolers. Little ones only know that something hurts, or that they can't see very well. The eye professional therefore needs to interact quietly with a child's parents as much as with the child to determine exactly what needs to be done.

Care for the infant starts, of course, during pregnancy. Expectant mothers should understand that drugs or alcohol are carried by the pregnant female's bloodstream directly to the fetus. Certain drugs may cause the child to suffer from drug addiction at birth and to suffer the shock of sudden drug withdrawal. In the case of alcohol, over-consumption may lead to *Fetal Alcohol Syndrome* (FAS). Even if FAS is not fatal, it still can have severe effects on the embryo, for it slows the rate of development of certain organs in the fetus, the eyes especially. The newborn infant on delivery will have eyes that are well below normal size. This tendency toward small, underdeveloped eyes will continue through childhood, and is not correctable.

The eyes of the newborn infant should be inspected immediately after birth by the pediatrician. Much can be learned about overall health, even at that early moment. The shape and position of the eyelids will frequently give the first indication of Down's syndrome, a problem most commonly found in mothers giving birth past 35 years of age. Slow pupillary reactions may suggest problems for the optic nerve.

A red eye or pink eye in the neonatal baby may indicate the presence of conjunctivitis or perhaps a potential or actual corneal ulcer. A chlamydial infection is not rare in neonatal infants and must be treated with antibiotics. If a discharge from the eyes continues past the neonatal period, it may be due to a congenital tear duct obstruction. In later infancy, there is a chance that fluid was pushed back into the conjunctival sac, causing the problem.

Continual, apparently unjustifiable eye movements of the neonatal infant, may indicate *nystagmus*. "Dancing eyes," an endless rocking or rotating of the eyes, can be produced by a tumor, an injury during birth, or a failure in early brain development. It may also reveal a congenital cataract which can be approached with infantile cataract surgery, muscular surgery, or glasses when the infant is old enough.

There is a reasonable chance a child may just outgrow nystagmus, unless a muscle imbalance sets in. It takes six weeks of life before the infant focuses and can relate his eyesight to information the brain has "filed" in order to permit meaningful vision. Prior to this time, about all that can be done by the doctor is to check the baby's ability to follow a light, or to evaluate pupillary reactions to stimuli.

Congenital blindness is quite rare. If an infant does not seem to react to light stimuli or to recognize his mother, and seems to follow sound instead of light, sophisticated tests can be given to examine the retina and the optic nerves (see Chapter Three).

A common practice is to place a premature infant in an oxygen-rich environment. This helps breathing while steps are being taken to increase the very low birth weight. While this is necessary to assure life, there may be a possibility of severe ophthalmic complications from the rich oxygen atmosphere referred to as *retinopathy of prematurity* (ROP), or the older term *retrolental fibroplasia* (RLF). With high oxygen, development of the retina's normal tiny veins and arteries is inhibited. When the oxygen is cut back, a rapid, almost uncontrollable development of blood vessels termed "neovascularizaton" begins. This can lead to retinal fibrosis, bleeding, shrinkage of the retina, or retinal detachment. The mass of scar tissue that develops in the place of a normal retina can easily lead to an irreversible blindness. Premature infants should therefore not be exposed to high oxygen any longer than is absolutely necessary. A very careful dilated retinal examination by a qualified ophthalmologist should be performed upon discharge or by two months of age. The best treatment is obstetrical prevention of premature births. This is not always possible. Mild cases often regress spontaneously. Advanced cases require special laser, cryopexy, and scleral buckling procedures. Success is very low in these cases. Your child will need to be checked carefully and often throughout his or her life.

Another uncommon, but serious eye disorder in newborn babies is the *congenital cataract*. This is possibly caused by the mother contracting measles early in pregnancy, or other prenatal problems. The congenital cataract is usually nuclear and complete. While the lens will become hard and solid after age 50 or 60, in the infant it is still quite flexible. The tissues holding the lens are very strong, making cataract extraction more difficult than for an adult. Meticulous care must be taken to remove as much lens material as possible because it is very toxic to the eye. Incomplete removals cause an intense inflammation to develop. Implanting an intraocular lens is not a good idea at this age unless the doctor is an experienced pediatric ophthalmologist, because the eye, like the rest of the child's body, is still growing. Any implant will soon be outgrown. The only practical solution may be to fit cataract eyeglasses and explain that when it is possible, a better solution will be applied. When the child is more mature, a contact lens may be utilized, epikeratophakia (see Chapter Eight) may be performed, or an intraocular lens may be implanted.

A condition which is relatively uncommon, but serious, is *infantile glaucoma,* with its attendant high intraocular pressure. The eye is a stretchable organ until the child reaches about three years of age, and a young child with chronic open-angle glaucoma may experience a marked growth of the elastic surface of the eye. This is

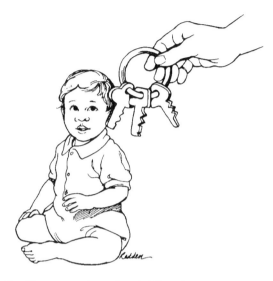

Figure 10–1   Please note how the child's right eye is turning inward, or is esotropic.

called *buphthalmos,* or "ox-eye," in which the eye becomes grotesquely larger than normal.

Other symptoms of glaucoma in the young, either congenital or infantile, are a high rate of tearing, and pain from exposure to light. Intraocular pressure usually must be measured under anesthesia shortly after the child falls asleep.

Muscle Imbalances

Strabismus, commonly known as "crossed eyes," refers to eyes that do not move together in a parallel fashion (Fig. 10–1). The eyes should turn right and left like the front wheels of a car, so that binocular focusing is possible. When they don't, it is due to a muscular imbalance in the six muscles, or a neurological disorder (Fig. 10–2A-C). Muscle imbalance that may be present at birth is usually noticed by a parent or pediatrician. The child should be seen by an ophthalmologist as soon as convenient.

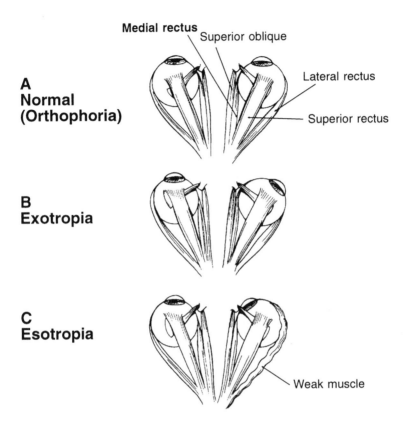

Figure 10–2 Muscular balance and muscular imbalance.
(A) Shows normal muscular balance. Please note both eyes are looking straight ahead.
(B) Shows a turning out of one eye, or exotropia.
(C) Shows a turning in of one eye, or esotropia. In this instance, the right lateral rectus is weak.

Crossed eyes often is first noticed in the very young when an infant's eyes react to a mobile hung above a crib or playpen. *Divergent strabismus,* or *exotropia,* is when one of the eyes moves or points outwardly on its own. If it tends to point toward the nose it is called *convergent strabismus,* or *esotropia.* Sometimes, most confusingly, both eyes may have a tendency to wander, producing the condition of *alternating strabismus*. This may be either permanent or temporary, but it is most likely to appear when the child is tired or sleepy. Partial paralysis of one of the eye muscles may cause *paralytic strabismus,* not treatable by the usual means to be described here.

The eye which is wandering or improperly focused transmits a blurred, vague, or double image to the brain from the retina (Fig. 10–3).

The brain has the ability to reject this confusing or faulty image and learns to accept only the clearer eye's image. To decrease confusion, the brain turns off the chemical conductors in the optic nerve so that the wandering eye is less able to transmit messages. Usually the child unconsciously stops using that eye, and if untreated, this leads to *amblyopia,* or "lazy eye." The result will be poor vision in that eye.

Children are neurologically distinctive compared to adults. *Ophthalmic maturity* is reached by age 10, and whatever levels of nerve function and ability to see are present by then are all that will ever be attained. Thus, all surgery, glasses, visual training, contact lenses, and the like are designed to have your child seeing as well as possible as he approaches and passes through the point of neurological maturation.

There is a tendency for strabismus, like glaucoma, to run in families. If any close relatives have had strabismus, watch for it in your own children.

When the eyes turn in the same direction, the paired muscles pull to the same degree in each eye, while the other pair of muscles both relax. The muscles are so positioned that the eyes can aim at any point within the same range. Each eye sees a target from a slightly different angle, as two minutely different pictures. The brain combines these pictures into one image through a process called *fusion* (Fig. 10–3A). It is the brain's comparison of the two slightly different views which permits focal triangulation, what we call depth perception.

But what if there is muscular imbalance? If one eye is looking directly at an object and the other eye is diverging away from it, the image transmitted from the locked-on-target eye

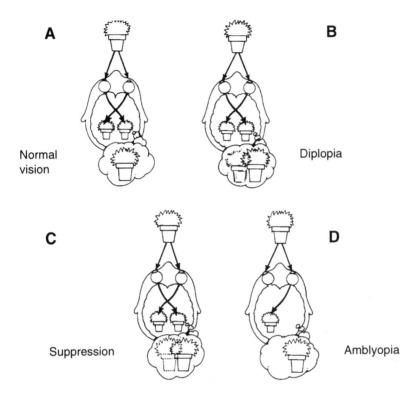

Figure 10–3 The progression of amblyopia.
(A) Normal "fusion" of the two eyes.
(B) Shows one eye turning out, causing double vision, or "diplopia."
(C) Shows the eye attempting to "suppress" the second image caused by the deviant eye.
(D) Total "suppression" of the second image, resulting in a blind, amblyopic eye.

will be concise, but the one from the other eye will be overlapping, producing a condition called *diplopia* (Fig. 10–3B). The brain tries to reconcile the images, but try as it may, the brain can't succeed. It learns to ignore the image sent by the wandering eye, either by suppressing it or by decreasing the intensity of the picture—"editing" it out (Fig. 10–3C). The wandering eye may be perfect in every other way, yet ignored. Unless this is corrected early on, the child will become permanently blind in the errant eye (Fig. 10–3D).

Fortunately, it is possible for the eye doctor to detect strabismus at a very early age. As an infant, the patterns of eye motion and focusing can be studied through simple tests, such as by watching the little one's eyes track objects. By age three, the child can be given a Snellen test using special charts. One might be a chart with large block capital E's. The examiner plays a game with the child, who is supposed to point his fingers in the same direction as the fingers of the E's on the chart. As an alternative, a vision chart may have little animals on it instead of letters, for children who don't yet know the alphabet.

An accurate examination of the eye's capacities is possible, if difficult. Holding a child so that dilating medicine can be dropped onto the eye can be the most trying part of the examination. After dilation, the doctor can look inside with an ophthalmoscope or gonioscope, or even attempt to measure intraocular pressure if there is the suspicion of infantile glaucoma.

The treatment and cure of strabismus is likely to require much time and patience on the part of the parents and the child. There are three routes possible. The first two, eyeglasses and patching, are preferred. Surgery is a last resort.

Glasses are prescribed if the eye examination has shown any significant refractive problems—nearsightedness, farsightedness, or severe astigmatism in the wandering eye. It sometimes happens that a refractive problem is all that is basically wrong with the child's eye wandering, simply because it cannot focus as well as its mate. Exercise of any muscle or organ tends to strengthen it, and powering up the problem eye so that it can focus may allow it to correct the undesirable tendency.

Prescribing eyeglasses for a young child is the easy part. Getting him to wear the glasses may require a program of motivations and penalties. If the eye is hyperopic, the glasses must be worn all the time. For a hyperopic child, the chances are good that the needed prescription will become weaker and weaker over a period of time until a point is reached when glasses may no longer be needed. If

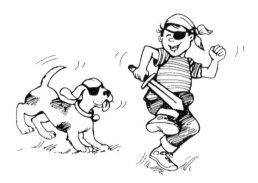

Figure 10-4 An example of how to make wearing an eye patch fun and successful.

glasses are prescribed, the shatter-proof polycarbonate type is best for active children. Contact lenses are very difficult for immature people to use, and their overuse—and the failure to perform important cleaning functions—can lead to disastrous infections.

If glasses fail to provide a solution, the ophthalmologist usually will choose prolonged treatment by patching. This means putting an eye patch on the good eye in order to force the child to use the wandering eye. If the patch is tight, and no visual cheating is possible, the procedure leaves no alternative but for the deviant eye to mend its ways.

The normal initial reaction of the child to a patch is to try to take it off. The child may be very obstinate about this. The way to approach matters is to set up a system of rewards for each day the patch is worn. Let the child color or decorate the patch. Work out some family games, like playing pirates in which other members of the family wears a similar patch. This may be hard to enforce on the family dog, but it's good for a laugh! The point is to make wearing the patch *fun* (Fig. 10-4).

For older children and special situations, contact lenses can be fitted. The contact lens on the weak eye is set to be as perfect as possible at distance. The good eye's contact is given too much power (over plussed) to see well near, hence the child can see perfectly nearby. The child is forced to use the weak eye to see far away. This works well and the stigma of the patch is bypassed.

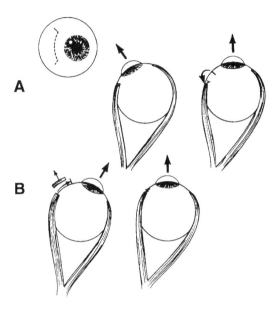

Figure 10–5   Techniques of muscle surgery.
(A) A procedure known as recession, where the muscle is cut and moved back.
(B) A procedure known as resection, where the length of the muscle is surgically shortened.

If, despite all efforts, there is no improvement in the strabismus the third choice is hospital surgery. When the child checks in, routine admittance tests are performed. Prior to the surgery, a relaxant is given to the child before he is anesthetized. An incision is made in the conjunctiva of the eye where the muscles are attached. If weakening is required, the muscle will be cut and moved further back on the sclera. This procedure is referred to as recession (Fig. 10–5A). If the muscle which poses a problem must be strengthened, the surgeon will remove a piece of muscle, reconnect the end, and suture this muscle back into place. This procedure is referred to as resection (Fig. 10–5B). The sutures are made using tiny stitches which will be absorbed by the body and do not have to be taken out after surgery. An eye patch may be placed over the closed post-op eye.

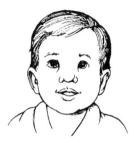

Figure 10–6 False strabismus, or "pseudostrabismus" which is common in young children. This condition is harmless and the child will outgrow it.

After the patch is removed and the eye has apparently returned to normal, a further examination is in order. The surgeon may find that an adequate muscular correction was not made and a further operation may be needed. Normally this is not the case but it can happen. Also, while the surgery may have aided in muscular correction, it may not have totally solved the strabismus, and a second round of patching, eyeglasses, or both may be needed.

One final thought. At the early stages of growth an extra width of skin across the bridge of the nose may cover the inner white scleral portion of the eye, making it appear that the eye is turned inward and that strabismus is present (Fig. 10–6). This condition is called "false strabismus" or "epicanthus." It is not a problem. The child will outgrow it as his facial features develop.

Children, especially the very young, cannot talk, and may be unaware that their eye condition is different than normal. Careful attention by family, pediatrician, and eye doctor is necessary to ensure good vision and muscle alignment.

Wrap-Up

- The appearance of squinting and excessive forced blinking in your child could signify the development of a refractive error. More often these observations are temporary habits or actions and disappear. A complete eye examination is indicated.

- Your neonatologist or pediatrician usually checks your baby's eyes soon after birth. You may ask to be sure. If your child was premature and oxygen supplementation to the incubator was required, a dilated retinal examination should be performed to check for possible retinopathy of prematurity (ROP).
- If there is no strong history of amblyopia, astigmatism, or strabismus in your family and your pediatrician evaluations seem normal, your child's first eye examination should be performed at preschool age.
- Your eye doctor should check your child again at approximately 12 to 14 years of age in early puberty.
- Ophthalmic maturity occurs at approximately age 10. All children need to be checked prior to this age for the presence of amblyopia. Extreme care to have the proper treatment, such as eyeglasses, contact lenses, patching of the eyes, or muscle surgery should be contemplated and ongoing during this developmental milestone to prevent amblyopia.
- If you notice a misalignment or improper eye positioning of your child's eyes, have your child evaluated.
- Shatterproof polycarbonate eyeglass lenses are best for active children and in sports situations.
- Ten percent of American children need visual correction.
- Among children with learning disabilities, only 10 percent have refractive errors requiring correction.

Chapter Eleven

Corneal and External Disease

Richard W. Yee and Deborah J. Yee

For those unaccustomed to thinking about such things, it comes as a surprise to learn that there are swarms of tiny organisms which surround our bodies at all times. In fact, these organisms live on us and inside us throughout our lives. They are so tiny that our eyes cannot see them, but they are there nonetheless. Most of the time they do not noticeably impair bodily functions and might as well not exist. It is only when a tiny organism creates an infection that its presence becomes evident and bothersome. Modern medicine approaches disease through a battery of mechanical, chemical, and radiation therapies.

It should come as no surprise that delicate organs such as the eyes and their supporting structures are especially vulnerable to disease. The eye area provides moisture, warmth, and the continuous exposure to the elements without the normal protection of skin cover. During sleep the interior systems of the eye are enveloped in gentle darkness one-fourth to one-third of the time. This provides a near-matchless environment in which an enterprising and aggressive microorganism can get rolling, should the body's natural defenses lower its guard for an instant.

Infections of the Eyelids

The subject of this chapter is the infection of the eye surfaces and neighboring tissues which confront the world most directly: the cornea and the eyelids. Eye problems have been recognized and studied by individuals interested in treating these problems since early time, as you learned in Chapter One. The effectiveness of treatment for superficial (but frequently serious!) eye diseases has progressed dramatically within the last two generations.

The various appearances and names of these infections are described by the special anatomical relationship of the eyelid organs. Each eyelid has a thick cartilage plate, known as the *tarsus*, along the margin which gives the eyelid shape, firmness, and structure.

Inflammation of the eyelids is still described in modern medicine with the ancient term *blepharitis*. "Blepharo" refers to the eyelashes. Blepharitis is usually caused by bacteria. This condition can become chronic because the many small glands involved in blepharitis have long, convoluted tubular ducts which hinder the drainage of thick infected material. Chronic blepharitis is equally difficult to treat because, in most instances, it is difficult or impossible to get sterilizing antibiotics up the small, swollen, convoluted tubules that are filled with infected materials.

Staphylococcal blepharitis is arguably the most common form of blepharitis, and is produced by the "staph" microorganisms which are always present on the eyelids. Staph microorganisms are usually contained by our immune systems. Ordinarily they do not create problems, but under certain circumstances these organisms can produce an infection of the eyelid margins, specifically the eyelash follicles. The infection usually spreads to adjacent sebaceous glands (Glands of Zeis) which open into the eyelash follicles. The eyelash follicles produce oily materials which keep our lashes soft and nonbrittle. The sweat glands of Moll empty into the lash follicles and also become filled with purulent material commonly called "pus." The tissue adjacent to these glands becomes necrotic, producing swollen, crusted eyelids that are tender and may bleed with the slightest trauma, even as gentle as warm compresses.

Patients with blepharitis who come into a clinic typically complain of such sensations as burning, irritation, itching, foreign body sensation, crusting in the corners of the eyes, and redness, especially upon awakening. The rims of their eyelids, or the "margins," may be red and inflamed.

Because the eyelash follicles are often infected, partial to total loss of the eyelashes may occur. The regrowth of eyelashes is a sign of positive response to treatment.

Seborrheic blepharitis occurs more often in those who have reached the high middle-age group, especially during and after the fifth decade of life. Sometimes it occurs simultaneously with staphylococcal blepharitis. Most patients who develop seborrheic blepharitis also have a skin condition called *seborrheic dermatitis,* identified by oily, "scaly" skin and inflammation of the scalp, eyebrows, nose, cheeks, top of the ears, or chest. In this disorder, the eyelid margins are red and oily scales form along the skin edge. When there are no associated bacterial organisms, *Pityrosporum ovale,* a yeast-like organism, can be seen under the microscope in material carefully scraped from the lid margin, but probably has little to do with the symptoms.

A localized purulent or suppurative infection of the eyelash follicle and of the glands of Zeis and Moll, usually caused by staphylococcus, is commonly called a *stye* or *external hordeolum.* These are usually tender, red, swollen lumps on the outside edge or front surface of the eyelid margin. These are acute inflammatory body responses to infection which tend to "point" to the inside surface of your eyelid.

Internal hordeolums are infections of the meibomian glands. Internal hordeolums can become *chalazions,,"* which is Greek for "lumps" (Fig. 11-1). Chalazions are chronic inflammatory responses, and are most common in the upper eyelids in both adults and children and are frequently associated with seborrheic and marginal blepharitis. The inflammation can be long-standing, yet sterile.

A chalazion results from chronic inflammation of the meibomian and/or Zeis glands. The infection breaks down the sebaceous (fat) producing cells of the glands. Since the glands are unable

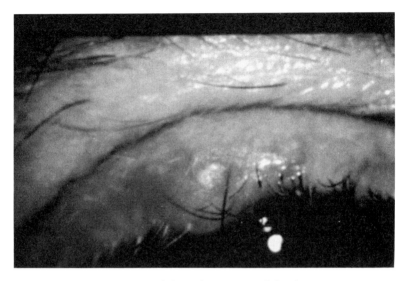

Figure 11–1   Chalazion of the right upper eyelid. This can cause pain, swelling, and redness.

to drain, the fat goes into the eyelid tissues, inciting an intense granulomatous response and forming a dense capsular wall or "gristle-like substance," as if you had a foreign body in your eyelid. As this chronic process develops, you will usually notice a painless "bump" in the eyelid. This is generally not at the edge of the eyelid, but away about 3/16 of an inch toward the eyelid fold.

The other possibility is an acute infection caused by the same organisms that produce blepharitis, producing an "acute chalazion." Chalazions may be small and unnoticeable, but they can also become a large lump on the eyelid, sometimes as large as one-half to three-quarters of an inch in diameter. At this scale, the lump is large enough to press on the eyeball and blur the vision. Tumors of the eyelids can mimic chalazions and must be kept in mind as a possibility when a "chalazion" does not resolve with treatment. Surgical alternatives vary widely and depend on the size and accessibility of the chalazion. Chalazions that are close to the lid margin can cause notching of the eyelid when removed, with a permanent loss of lashes.

Should the body be unable to seal off the bacteria and associated gland secretions, the eyelid and surrounding eye tissues may rapidly become infected. This *orbital cellulitis* is potentially fatal and demands immediate attention because the venous drainage from around the eye flows backward around the base of the brain.

The diagnosis and treatment of these different conditions is the same in many ways. First, your doctor will take a history. Then he will examine your eyes with and without the high magnification slit lamp biomicroscope. The diagnosis frequently is obvious and the physician will begin your care immediately. When necessary, eyelid cultures and scrapings analyses are performed in the lab to verify the diagnosis.

Treatment of staph blepharitis involves long-term, careful attention to the eyelid and personal hygiene, as well as use of antibiotics. The frequency and length of treatment depends upon the severity of the infection. Hot compresses should be used as often and as long as possible. Generally this means a small hand towel soaked with hot water from the faucet applied to your eye, changing it often to keep the contact warm to hot. Moist towels are far superior to a "dry heat" heating pad. Many minor problems will be cured by hot compresses, and further treatment will usually be unnecessary.

You should use an antibiotic soap when washing your face. In our study, 89 percent of the patients who had developed infections had not been using deodorant soaps. Special attention about cleaning and debriding dead cells and discharge materials from the eyelashes is needed. Baby shampoo diluted three-to-one with water, or over-the-counter eyelid scrub agents such as Eye-Scrub™ or Ocuclenz™, applied with cotton tipped applicators or the soft cotton squares found in pharmacy cosmetic displays, can be used. Scrub the eyelid gently each morning to remove the accumulations from the previous night's sleep.

Your doctor also will prescribe antibiotic eyedrops. Follow instructions carefully and use the eyedrops in *both* eyes (unless otherwise instructed by your doctor) since the bacteria is generally present in both eyes. You may be given ointment salves such as bacitracin or erythromycin to put in each eye at bedtime. More severe or chronic cases of infection may also require administration of oral antibiotics for weeks or even months.

It is important to understand that once your eyelids are infected and scarring occurs, you may never be totally cured. More accurately, the problem can be kept under control. If seborrhea is discovered on the scalp or other skin surfaces, part of the treatment probably should involve discussing overall hygiene with a patient. Encouraging regular washing with deodorant soaps and shampoos containing anti-seborrheal agents can make dramatic results possible on occasion. These soaps should be applied full-strength to the scalp, around the ears, eyebrows, sideburns, and on the sides of the nose and allowed to remain 10 to 30 minutes. Rinse off in the shower and repeat one to three times a week as needed, and seborrhea will be contained.

Pressure and discomfort in some local pockets of infection may require drainage to encourage healing and relief from pain. This is usually accomplished by "pricking" under topical anesthesia, using a small, thin surgical knife or surgical needle. After drainage, matters should resolve in several days.

If orbital cellulitis develops, use of intense oral and possibly intravenous antibiotics may be necessary. In small children and in some adults, immediate hospitalization might be a good idea.

Sometimes, injections of a steroid may be recommended, or even surgical removal of the lumps. Steroid injections have the disadvantage of sometimes causing hypopigmentation and atrophy over the area of treated skin.

In cases where the eyelid infection does not resolve in a reasonable amount of time and the inflammation continues to flourish, the doctor may choose to take a tiny piece of tissue for lab analysis to culture the tissue and to rule out the possibility of a tumor. This sounds tricky and painful, not to mention the likelihood of producing a scar, but that is not the case. Tissue sampling or biopsy is easy and leaves only the slightest lingering sign of the biopsy visible under the microscope. If a tumor is present, some variety of chemotherapy, radiation treatment, or surgery may be advisable. Otherwise, the doctor will probably culture or reculture the eyelids and continue his exploration of medications to find which one will work.

Infections of the Conjunctiva

Conjunctivitis, also known either as "red eye" or "pinkeye," is an inflammation of the conjunctiva, the very thin membrane-like mucous membrane that produces fluids which coat and lubricate the surface of the eye. When the conjunctiva becomes irritated or inflamed, this membrane and its associated blood vessels become more prominent and the eye turns red and sticky.

There are all sorts of conjunctivitis. Biological vectors— bacteria, viruses, fungi, and parasites—hold the lead in causing conjunctivitis, but the modern world offers a multitude of other possible means of developing this disease. Airborne exposure to environmental irritants can cause allergy of the mucous membrane referred to as *allergic conjunctivitis,* as can drug reactions, contact with foreign bodies, chemical sprays, preservatives in contact lens solutions, and other irritants. Often it is difficult to diagnose a cause and an ophthalmologist who has special training in corneal and external diseases may need to be consulted. In the temperate climates of the world, where most of the modern technologically advanced societies reside, visitors returning from the tropics may exhibit conjunctivitis produced by exotic agents known only to a few theoretical researchers and rarely seen in the civilized world.

Whatever the cause, conjunctivitis causes the eye to become very irritated and red. The eye may presently begin to be painful or overly light-sensitive. There may be tearing and a sticky discharge which, when dried out overnight, will cause the eyelids to stick together in the morning. This can be startling, especially to young children experiencing it for the first time. However, the type of discharge is helpful in analyzing possible biological or other culprits producing the flow. The doctor may scrape the conjunctiva with a cotton swab so that evaluation in the lab can determine the cause. If a test is positive for a set of microorganisms, sometimes cultures with antibiotic sensitivity are worked up before treatment is begun. The doctor will also make certain that the cornea and iris are not infected and that there has been no increase in intraocular pressure.

Typical treatment of conjunctivitis begins immediately, on general principles. While laboratory results are out, topical and sometimes systemic antibiotic treatment can be started. If this does not help after several days, a combination of steroid and antibiotic drops may be started with careful monitoring, especially in the case of steroids. If this does not work and the lab results are back, then a careful reevaluation and review of other causes begins.

If the cause is a virus, antibiotic treatment is ineffective and the disease, like a cold, must run its course. In *viral conjunctivitis* a watery discharge is present and lasts from one to two weeks. Viruses are often associated with a sore throat, a runny nose, and also sneezing. Therefore, viral conjunctivitis is highly contagious and spreads with remarkable ease to anyone who comes within close range.

Conjunctivitis caused by allergies is fairly easy to identify and treat. Some allergies are related to hay fever and make the eyes red and itchy. Others just produce a chronic irritation and redness. Treatment of this form of conjunctivitis obviously means attempting to remove or diminish contact with environmental irritants, such as smoke fumes or pollen that cause the conjunctivitis. Topical nonsteroidal anti-inflammatory drugs such as Acular™, mast cell stabilizers like Alomide™, antihistamines such as Livostin™, vasoconstrictors and ice compresses are effective in helping sufferers from allergic conjunctivitis.

Corneal Injuries

In the course of daily life, minor injuries to the eye are common. The cornea is especially subject to bruises or scratches, particularly the outermost layer of the cornea, the corneal epithelium. Causes can include contact lenses, a baby's fingernail, a paper cut, tree limbs or bushes, a head-on collision between hypermacho young football players, even vigorous rubbing of the eye. Certain corneal conditions such as dry eyes, some of the corneal dystrophies, and any irritation of the cornea can contribute to this type of injury.

Because the cornea contains many pain nerve fibers, the most significant symptom in this sort of condition is severe, immediate pain. Other symptoms to look for are watery eyes and light sensitivity. There is usually no pus-like discharge unless the corneal damage has fostered a secondary bacterial infection. Although an abrasion may be in only one eye, the other eye may also become sensitive to light and show the same symptomatic response of excess tearing.

In addition to pain and light sensitivity, an observant onlooker may notice that the injured person frequently squeezes the eyelids in an attempt to ease the pain. Because this pain is so excruciating, it may be difficult for a doctor to examine a patient. Often a drop of anesthetic solution can momentarily give enough time for a quick but adequate eye examination. The doctor will usually use the yellow dye called fluorescein to determine the extent of the injury to the epithelium. An antibiotic ointment is typically put into the eye after that, and an eye bandage with firm and gentle pressure is placed over the eye to prevent the eyelids from moving over the injured area.

The anesthetic drops are not given for pain at this point because they slow the eye's epithelium from healing properly if used over and over again. Certain new non-steroidal anti-inflammatory drops and pills generally do an excellent job of reducing and relieving the pain. A drug that will relax the spasming of the eye (cycloplegic agent) will also aid in improving comfort. It is important to have daily re-examinations of the eye so that infection or ulcer formation can be spotted early. Usually there is quick improvement as the pain, light sensitivity factor, and watery discharge decrease.

A corneal erosion or abrasion will heal in two to three days, depending on the extent of the injury. Curiously, after an abrasion heals, it can spontaneously return, and is usually noticed upon awakening. When this *recurrent erosion* occurs, it is because the attachments of the newly healed epithelium are not firmly attached to the tissue below. Repeated patching, use of ointments at bedtime, and a soft bandage contact lens or collagen shield—a contact lens made of protein that dissolves after a few days—may be necessary. Fortunately, most corneal abrasions heal without any problems at all.

Corneal Dystrophies

A "corneal dystrophy" is a degeneration of the cornea. Luckily for all of us, it is a rare group of disorders. For descriptive purposes, corneal dystrophies are broken down into several groups, identified by where the abnormalities are found in the three layers of the cornea: the epithelium, the stroma, and the endothelium. They are characterized by being bilateral (in both eyes), slowly progressive, degenerative, and hereditary with unknown cause. They are usually associated with abnormal deposits of substances that alter the normal corneal architecture. These substances can interfere with your vision and make the corneal surface painful. The dystrophies usually develop during the first or second decade, but in some cases appear later in life, such as *Fuchs' dystrophy*. Most corneal dystrophies are stationary, in other words stabilized, but some are slowly progressive. If your vision decreases seriously, a corneal transplant may be suggested. The only trouble is that because this is a hereditary disorder, recurrences of the dystrophy can and do happen regularly in the newly grafted cornea, producing the same problem in spite of all efforts to the contrary.

Another epithelial dystrophy is called *anterior epithelium basement membrane dystrophy* and is sometimes called *map-dot-fingerprint dystrophy,* or *Cogan's microcystic dystrophy*. It occurs simultaneously in both eyes. During an examination, a doctor will notice various patterns of dots, lines, and irregularities on the epithelium of the cornea. It occurs more commonly in women after age 40. Most patients do not show symptoms, but some notice a foreign body sensation and blurring of the vision. Recurrent episodes of tissue breakdown are moderately common, typically occurring in the morning when the patient awakes with very sharp, stabbing pain. Treatment for this condition is similar to the treatment of a corneal abrasion.

Corneal stromal dystrophies are an inherited condition, and involve the excessive production of some abnormal products in the cells that make up the stromal layer of the cornea. The accumulation of these deposits may cause no symptoms or may cause significant visual impairments. Most can be treated with surgery, ranging from a removal of the corneal surface (lamellar keratectomy) to a corneal transplant.

Corneal Edema

Corneal edema (also called *bullous keratopathy, epithelial edema,* and *stromal edema*) is the term for excess water in the cornea. This situation is produced when the balance between the forces driving water into the cornea and those pushing water out is upset.

In the normal eye, pressure inside the eye tends to force fluid into the cornea. The front surface of the cornea is protected from absorbing water from the tears by the water barrier function of some of the corneal layers. The water in the cornea is removed as a normal metabolic function of the endothelial cells on the inside of the cornea and through evaporation into the air from the front surface of our cornea. If anything goes out of balance, fluid build-up in the cornea will produce increased corneal depth. Patients complain of blurred vision that is more severe in the morning and improves as the day progresses. As the fluid pressure worsens, small cysts on the epithelium may burst open, producing sharp, stabbing pains, light sensitivity, and redness. If untreated, continual attacks of this edema will cause scarring of Bowman's membrane and the stroma. There will also be a markedly increased chance that blood vessels will grow into the cornea, influencing the amount and character of light which can enter the eye.

Many hereditary diseases of the endothelium can cause corneal fluids to build up to an unhealthy degree. Some appear at birth, others in mature adults. For example, Fuchs' endothelium dystrophy, which occurs later in life, can be diagnosed by using a slit lamp biomicroscope to identify many small elevated bumps on the endothelial layer just behind the Descemet's membrane. These are called *corneal guttata*. Fuchs' is much more common in women than in men, for unknown reasons.

The endothelium can be damaged by disease. Another source of injury is intraocular surgery if there is contact with surgical instruments. Whenever there is a disruption of Descemet's membrane, the aqueous humor can enter the cornea and cause edema. Typically, the endothelial cells will grow over the wound and heal the membrane, decreasing the edema over several months. A scar can remain after one of these episodes.

There are other possible sources of damage to the endothelium. The very drugs, preservatives, and irrigating solutions used during surgery can set off an adverse reaction and damage it. Intruding blood, high intraocular pressures, contact lenses (which induce starvation of oxygen to the corneal endothelium if improperly worn), and inflammation can also damage the endothelial barrier and permit the occurrence of corneal edema. Inflammation of the internal structures of the eye, known as *anterior uveitis,* can be painful and cause visual impairment and blindness. The endothelium can become attacked by the cells of the immune system, allowing excess fluid to enter the cornea. Certain organisms, such as *herpes simplex* and *herpes zoster,* can produce the same effect. An inflammation may come about after a corneal transplant during graft rejection where lymphocytes migrate into the graft, destroying helpless endothelial cells which happen to be in the way.

When corneal edema is a problem, agents which pull the water from the cornea can be used. A two percent to five percent salt-water solution draws the water out of the cornea and moderates the visual blurring caused by the edema. These drops should be given more frequently in the morning because retention of fluid is greatest immediately upon awakening. A five percent salt ointment may be beneficial at bedtime, or even such a mundane alternative as aiming a hairdryer at arm's length at the cornea to increase evaporation of the corneal surface.

Microcysts in the cornea that are not inherited can occur after epithelium wound healing and in patients who have had an injury to the cornea, who are long-standing contact lens wearers or who have experienced toxicity from chronic use of topical ocular agents. These cysts tend to decrease your vision, cause pain and irritation, and cause significant light sensitivity. Treatment generally involves eliminating the causative agent listed above.

In advanced cases of corneal fluid build-up where there are microcysts and bullae (blisters), drops can be used to relax eye muscle spasm and aid the patient's comfort. Nonsteroidal anti-inflammatory medication taken by mouth, such as Ansaid™, may also be prescribed, to effectively relieve. Soft contact lenses can be prescribed to provide a smooth, protective surface for

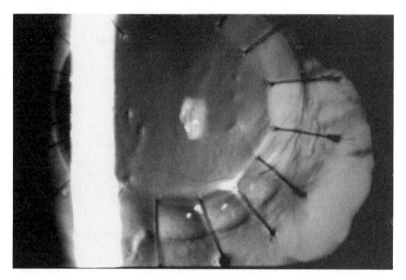

Figure 11–2 "Slit lamp" photograph of a clear graft or "corneal transplant" sutured with many fine microsurgical sutures.

the cornea. This may also relieve complaints of a foreign body sensation caused by microcysts.

Corneal Transplants

Corneal transplants have become the modern treatment of choice to improve vision caused by irreversible corneal edema (Fig. 11–2). A corneal transplant surgery can be performed along with a lens extraction, and with or without implanting a new lens when indicated. By the same token, patients who have already had their natural lens removed can have a corneal transplant and get an artificial lens implant at the same time. The success rate of corneal transplantation for corneal edema is very good, but potential vision afterward may be limited depending on how well the retina functions. In patients who have painful, light sensitive bullae with no potential for vision after corneal surgery, use of a small mucous membrane flap from the conjunctiva to cover the cornea, or cauterization in the cornea, may eliminate the pain caused by the ruptured bullae. If advanced corneal fluid build-up is not treated, a patient very likely will feel chronic pain and irritation, and there will always be the possibility of secondary infection. Early treatment for these conditions is a good idea.

Corneal Ulcers

Corneal ulcers, or open sores, can produce a terrifying "melting away" of the cornea. They are caused by infection with bacteria, viruses, fungi, and the invasion of certain parasites. Direct encounters with toxic chemicals, like an accidental spray of Drano™, can cause ulcer-like destruction of tissue. Because corneal ulcers are a sight-threatening process, and it is difficult to separate infectious causes from other types of ulcerative and infiltrative processes, careful microbiological and chemical evaluation is necessary for each case.

When a corneal ulcer develops, patients frequently may have the feeling that there is something in their eye. The eye may become red, painful, light-sensitive, experience decreased vision, and produce a pus-like discharge. Your doctor may notice only mild, localized whitening of the cornea which will stain with fluorescein staining. These localized areas of grayish whitening may be shallow or deep, depending upon how severe the ulceration has become (Fig. 11–3). During an initial examination, the doctor sketches a detailed drawing of the ulcer. It shows the ulcer's size, shape, and the amount of stromal involvement. A photograph may be taken to document its appearance. Because the ulceration could be caused by inflammation and have no relation to biological infectious causes, it is necessary to take corneal scrapings for thorough lab analysis. In addition, it may be a good idea to take material with a cotton-tip swab from the ulcer, the lid margins, and conjunctiva for the same sort of lab work.

Since time is of the essence, while the lab is studying the samples, treatment begins with antimicrobial drops known to hinder or kill a broad spectrum of organisms. These drops may be given every half hour to every hour during the first 24 to 48 hours after the first examination. Certain severe ulcerations may warrant antibiotic in-

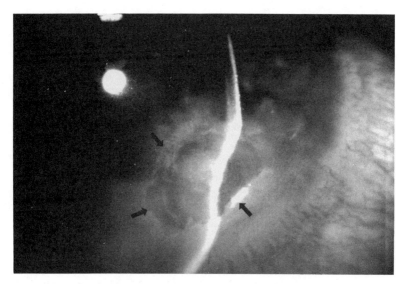

Figure 11-3 "Slit lamp" photograph of a corneal ulcer. The corneal ulcer is of moderate depth near the periphery of the cornea.

jections under the mucous membrane covering of the eye, the subconjunctival spaces. Medications given either orally or intravenously could be necessary for ulcerations that extend to the white of the eye, or if there is pending or existing corneal perforation.

Modification of this treatment depends on the patient's response to the initial therapy and what was found on the corneal scrapings and/or cultures. Improvement is closely monitored by frequent examinations. If the corneal ulcer continues to enlarge even in the context of therapy, it is not uncommon to repeat scrapings and cultures. Hospitalization with sedation is sometimes necessary if a patient does not feel competent to administer his own medication.

Corneal ulceration can also be produced by some rather unexpected mechanisms such as dry eye syndromes, unconscious rubbing of the eye while asleep, melting from rheumatoid arthritis, or corneas that have lost their sensation (*neurotrophic ulcers*). People can cause ulceration themselves through inadequate knowledge and the unsupervised use of anesthetic drops, which cause the cornea to become desensitized and block the reproduction of the epithelial cells, subsequently causing melting and ulceration.

Dry Eyes

Dry eyes is a common and peculiarly uncomfortable condition, and since this dryness can cause so many problems it deserves some discussion. Recalling the nature of how tear films are formed, note also that certain conditions of the eyelid like entropion (when the eyelid turns in), ectropion (when the eyelid turns out), or lagophthalmos (incomplete closure of the eyelid) can cause the tear film to spread incompletely on the eye surface, causing dry spots and, therefore, a dry eye. There is a lot more to it than just this, unfortunately.

Frequently, patients with dry eyes complain early in the disease of burning and a scratchy or sandy foreign body sensation. These symptoms are usually worse at the end of the day than at the beginning, in contrast to blepharitis symptoms. Other symptoms include itching, excessive mucus secretion, inability to produce tears, burning sensation, increased photosensitivity, redness, pain, or a heaviness or difficulty in moving the eyelid. The doctor may detect a decreased volume of tears in the eyes. There may be some redness, and the conjunctiva may seem a little bit parched.

In more severe diseases, there may be strands of mucus attached to the cornea and areas of melting. Patients with dry eyes may also complain of increased tearing, because when the eye becomes dry, it tells the brain that dryness is occurring and the brain, as a physiological response, produces more tears and causes the excess tearing even though the eye remains dry in spots. These are sometimes called "reflex tears."

By using filter paper strips placed just inside the lower eyelid, the degree of tear production can be measured. The use of rose bengal staining may help to diagnose dry eyes early so that the condition will not be missed by using just a slit lamp without the dye. Depending on the severity of the condition, certain blood tests can help diagnose some of the diseases that are associated with dry eye syndromes.

Treatment depends on the cause of dry eyes. In most early cases, treatment with over-the-counter artificial tears is used to lubricate and replace the inadequate tear film. There are many different brands of artificial tears, and the individual should try several to determine the most beneficial brands. Generally, preservative-free products are better.

There are two draining duct openings in each of the eyes, and sometimes the doctor will consider some degree of blocking the drainage temporarily or permanently. This blockage keeps the tears in the eye for a longer period of time, resulting in moister eyes and greater eye comfort, especially during the winter time. Staying away from air conditioning and heater vents, which produce dry air, is wise. There are also devices that can be put around the eyeglasses to cut down on the evaporation of the tears due to wind.

Surgery is sometimes necessary if the eyes are severely dry. Partial, temporary, or permanent closure of a portion or the entire eyelid, called "tarsorrhaphy," may be necessary. If there is an associated melting of the cornea due to extreme dryness, corneal transplantation combined with tarsorrhaphy and/or a conjunctival flap may be necessary. These conditions are usually associated with severe systemic diseases such as rheumatoid arthritis.

Excessive Tearing

Dry eyes can cause damage to the cornea. Excessive tearing, or *epiphora,* can produce excessive wiping of tears, not to mention exasperation. Such tearing can be associated with pain, emotional distress, or eye irritation caused by some reflex stimulation like eye strain, corneal injury, or a foreign body on the cornea. Tearing can also be caused by yawning, vomiting, and excessive laughing. Epiphora can follow blockage of the tear drainage system, and may also result from conditions such as congenital glaucoma with a cloudy cornea, and high fluid pressures in the eyes. Lastly, certain environmental conditions such as wind, pollen, or smoke can irritate the eyes and cause tearing.

If the cause of epiphora is due to complete or partial closure of the nasolacrimal duct from birth, then several weeks of massaging the tear sac, located near the inner corner of the eye, and antibiotic drops may be recommended. *Canaliculitis,* which is an infection of a portion of the drainage pathway, needs to be treated with the appropriate antibiotics. The disease may necessitate surgery. Infections of the lacrimal sac called *dacryocystitis,* are managed by topical ophthalmic and systemic antibiotics. This condition, if not improved by medical treatment, may need to be resolved by dacryocystorhinostomy (DCR), where an opening is made from the lacrimal sac into the nose.

Surgical treatment for epiphora, again like medical treatment, necessitates adequate diagnosis before removing any local irritating disorders, such as eyelashes rubbing on the cornea or malpositioning of the eyelids. For the lacrimal pump to work effectively, the lid must be in proper position so that the tears will drain appropriately into the lacrimal drainage system. Sometimes the drainage openings or "puncta" are too small or are not in the correct position. The puncta can be opened surgically to correct an anatomical or physiological spastic "closure." If this does not work, sometimes a silicone tube needs to be placed in the tear duct. When the canaliculus is completely closed or absent, then a direct opening into the lacrimal sac is made. When the nasolacrimal duct system is blocked from birth, thin rods of different sizes that fit into and open the drainage system offer an excellent cure rate.

Episcleritis and Scleritis

Episcleritis is an inflammation of the Tenon's capsule, which lies between the conjunctiva and the sclera. The sclera itself may or may not be inflamed. If it is inflamed, the disease is called *scleritis.* It is important for your eye doctor to distinguish between the two. Episcleritis is usually a benign, self-healing, and easily treated condition. Scleritis, however, can be destructive and cause blindness if left untreated. The cause of episcleritis is unknown. It is more common in females than males, and usually occurs after age 40.

Initially in episcleritis, a patient may notice redness over the entire eye or just a portion of the eye. Slight pain, light sensitivity, tenderness, and increased tearing are usual complaints. In addition, inflammatory nodules or bumps may be present. Mild inflammation of the front chamber of the eye is not uncommon. Because episcleritis is self-limiting, it usually produces no damage to the eye and requires no treatment. In certain cases that linger or are associated with pain, anti-inflammatory agents or topical steroids may be applied. If an apparent case of episcleritis does not resolve itself, it may be important to rule out other diseases that cause inflammation, such as collagen vascular diseases.

Scleritis, a much more serious matter, is deceptive. It may look very much like an ordinary case of episcleritis when much more is afoot. Because scleritis is the inflammation of the sclera, which is composed of collagen, it is frequently associated with diseases of the body that involve collagen—like rheumatoid arthritis, systemic lupus erythematous, and other connective tissue diseases.

The patient notices the symptoms as seen in episcleritis, except that there may be considerably more pain and light sensitivity, and the front chamber of the eye may be a good deal more inflamed. The cornea can be also inflamed. Although most of the inflammation is in the front portions of the eye, it can spread to the back of the eye and involve the optic nerve and retina. Lab tests to verify this condition may nearly include the kitchen sink: a complete blood count, erythrocyte sedimentation rate, uric acid level, syphilis serology, plasma protein electrophoresis, rheumatoid factor, antinuclear antibody, and possibly chest and sacroiliac X-rays. Your eye doctor may also want you to see a specialist in arthritic conditions.

The treatment for scleritis usually includes anti-inflammatory agents, which may include the non-steroidal inflammatory agents such as flubiprofen or indocin. Steroids are sometimes necessary in severe cases that do not respond to initial medication. Immunosuppressive agents, like cyclophosphamide, could be prescribed. Because scleritis might be the first warning of underlying systemic connective tissue problems, it is important to continue treatment with a rheumatologist or internist. In some cases, long-term treatment lasting for months or years is necessary to control the inflammation.

Herpetic Infections

Herpes zoster is a viral disease that causes a skin rash that may start as little red dots that become fluid-filled blisters which form scabs and may leave significant scars. This is the same virus that is associated with the chickenpox seen in childhood. The virus lingers on in the body's cells, and can become active again in later life when the immune system is weakened for some reason, as in aging. The virus usually attacks along the region of the skin which is supplied by nerves. In herpes zoster, the virus infects the nerve system that informs one side of the upper portion of the face. If the virus infects the nerves that supply the eye, it can not only cause the skin rash but a corneal inflammation, ulcers, anterior chamber reaction, and subsequent increases in the fluid pressure of the eye. Sometimes, because the nerves are injured during this infection's course, there may be some mild to severe pain which remains for years after the initial infection.

You may first notice some mild itching to severe pain over one side of the face, usually involving the forehead and the eyelids. There may be decreased vision with redness, increased tearing, and discharge in the involved eye. Double vision can occur in some cases. It is important for your doctor to do a complete examination to rule out any involvement of the cornea, extraocular muscles, retina, and optic nerve. No diagnostic tests are usually necessary except to rule out associated diseases such as certain cancers, i.e. lymphoma, or particularly in young people, the seemingly ubiquitous HIV viruses.

This disease is usually treated with acyclovir, or other antiviral medications. In treating the ocular side of herpes zoster, topical steroids are helpful in decreasing the amount of inflammation. Topical antibiotics may also be applied to prevent secondary infection. Because there is a decrease in corneal sensation, a bandage lens may be necessary to encourage healing and to prevent corneal melting. It is important to know that recurrences of ocular herpes zoster can occur even after the rash is gone. Long-term checkup visits with the diagnosing doctor are essential.

Herpes simplex is a virus that can infect the skin, the mucous membranes of the mouth, the sex organs, and the eye. There are two major types of herpes simplex virus. Herpes simplex type one is most common and is usually responsible for diseases that are above the beltline, including eye diseases and the more common cold sore or fever blister that can occur on the face. Type two is the sexually transmitted herpes virus which rarely causes diseases above the waist, but is not unknown among the more sexually adventurous.

Herpetic infections around the eye are usually minor. There may be simply formations of small blisters on the skin of the eyelids, or you may notice only mild irritation and light sensitivity. If the cornea becomes infected, some blurred vision may be noticed. After the primary infection, always the worst instance, recurrent infection is usually in the form of an ulceration of the cornea called *dendritic keratitis*. In addition to having a red eye, there may be an associated anterior chamber inflammation or scleral inflammation. It is also possible for the retina to be infected, but this is very rare. Many times a doctor will not take a culture because the appearance of the eye with this infection is very characteristic. It is important to ensure that no bacterial infection creeps in to enjoy a weakened immune system and the opportunities offered by an open ulcer.

The initial treatment of herpes simplex epithelial disease includes antiviral eye medications such as trifluorothymidine (Viroptic™). Other topical antiviral agents include iodoxuridine and vidarabine. At first, these are applied every hour while you are awake, then they are slowly tapered off as the situation improves. A topical eye muscle relaxant is often used to decrease the amount of light sensitivity and spasm of the ciliary muscle. No steroids should be prescribed in the treatment of herpetic epithelial keratitis. If a secondary bacterial infection is suspected, a topical antibiotic drug may also be necessary. Topical corticosteroids are never given in active epithelium disease, but may be necessary in cases with stromal and disciform herpetic disease as the eye becomes more quiet.

Corneal melting and perforation can occur in very severe herpetic eye involvement, and even the secondary scarring may produce effects which are uncomfortable. "Gluing" with a tissue glue may be necessary in preparation for corneal transplanting. An eye surgeon may wish to wait until the eye is quiet and without recurrent disease before considering this procedure. Most people only experience the initial episode of herpes simplex, but 25 percent of people who have a corneal infection are likely to have another infection within two years.

Keratoconus

Keratoconus is a corneal disorder where the central cornea becomes thin and protrudes in a cone-shaped fashion. The cause of keratoconus is unknown and does not display a specific pattern of inheritance. The disease usually begins in adolescence and may affect one or both eyes. The most early complaints include blurring and distortion of vision, perhaps along with a history of astigmatism, frequent changes in glasses, or an inability to wear hard contact lenses. Keratoconus occurs equally in men and women and, if any correlation can be made for it, seems slightly more associated with people who have allergies on the skin, asthma, a history of eye rubbing, Down's syndrome, or Leber's congenital amaurosis. Certain specialized tests, such as corneal topography analysis, can help diagnose keratoconus by spotting the corneal steepening. Keratoconus has been successfully treated with glasses or contact lenses. A corneal transplant is necessary when the patient can no longer wear contact lenses, or if vision with contact lenses is no longer satisfactory. Transplants in keratoconus are quite successful but there are associated risks of rejecting the graft, developing a cataract, glaucoma, or developing an irregular corneal surface.

Subconjunctival Hemorrhage

Subconjunctival hemorrhage is simply the collection of blood underneath the mucous membrane layer of the eye. This commonly develops without any specific cause, and usually in one eye. There is no age correlation, and typically no associated symptoms. Suddenly the eye becomes bright red, quite an alarming situation. The hemorrhage is caused by a rupture of a small conjunctival vessel. The physician will typically notice bright red blood underneath the conjunctiva on slit lamp examination. This bright red patch of blood can begin to spread and settle with gravity during the next several days. If the bleeding is heavy, then the blood may eventually become dark red. As the blood breaks down, it changes to look like a bruise.

While most subconjunctival hemorrhages are caused by a blood vessel breaking due to rubbing the eye, a history of injuries, infection, vomiting, coughing, constipation, diabetes, hematologic diseases and hypertension can each be a potential culprit aiding and abetting. Encounters with chemicals can be associated directly with subconjunctival hemorrhage, or may indirectly cause it by irritating the eye and causing the individual to rub the eye too vigorously, producing the hemorrhage. It is not uncommon to see subconjunctival hemorrhage after ocular surgery. In most cases, the hemorrhage will usually be reabsorbed after two or three weeks.

Pterygium and Pinguecula

Pterygium (Fig. 11-4) is an unsightly abnormal growth on the surface of the eye which may or may not interfere with vision. The pterygium is a fleshy, typically wedge-shaped growth that may be elevated and extends toward the center of the cornea. The exact cause of a pterygium is not well understood, but a fairly conclusive theory is that it is associated with long-term exposure to ultraviolet sunlight and chronic irritation from dry, dusty conditions. Pterygia develop more in people who spend a great deal of time outdoors exposed to sun, wind, and dust. A pterygium is usually nothing but a bother, but it can cause itching, burning, and scratchiness. Squamous cell carcinoma and a pterygium have a similar appearance. During periods of growth, the pterygium will cause a red eye. Vision loss can occur if the pterygium grows over the cornea and causes astigmatism problems. The growth usually occurs on the nasal side of the eye, but not always. Because the pterygium is elevated, it may cause areas of dryness on the cornea which are called *dellen*.

When a pterygium becomes irritated, topical lubricants, non-steroidal anti-inflammatory agents, or vasoconstrictor drops may help reduce the inflammation. If the pterygium is large enough to threaten sight, or it is growing or is cosmetically too unsightly, it

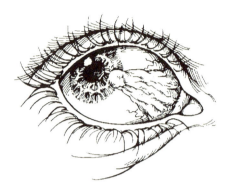

Figure 11–4   Pterygium is fibrovascular growth over and beyond the limbus onto the clear cornea.

can be removed surgically. Recurrences are common in young people. Sometimes radiation treatment and certain topical medications can be used to help decrease this possibility. Protecting the eyes from ultraviolet light with proper sunglasses, and avoiding dry, dusty environments may also be helpful.

A *pinguecula* (Fig. 11–5) is a thickening, or lump, of the conjunctiva beside the eye, more commonly on the nasal side. It can appear as a yellowish or white lesion and is composed of benign, fat-like degenerated tissue. A pinguecula is different from a pterygium in that it never grows onto the cornea.

Causes of a pinguecula are similar to the causes of a pterygium. It is thought to be common in people who spend a large part of their lives outdoors in sunny, dusty, sandy, and windy environments. Many people with pingueculae have no complaints, but when one eye becomes inflamed, there may be some burning or stinging. It may become red and irritated, and quite unsightly. If this happens, hot compresses, vasoconstrictor and/or steroid eyedrops may be used to clear the redness and irritation. Most of the time these growths do not interfere with vision and in most cases there is no need for treatment, unless it is cosmetically necessary.

Most of us take our vision and health for granted. One of my corneal transplant patients who was born with poor corneas and vision shares her thanks and in so doing keeps us mindful. She cried

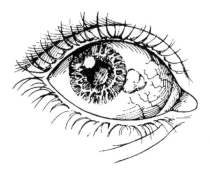

Figure 11-5   Pinguecula is usually an amber to yellowish elevated growth adjacent to the cornea.

when she saw the lace on her gown for the first time. Each visit was another observation — "I saw clouds for the first time" and "leaves on trees" and most recently "rain drops!" These are precious reminders to each of us.

Corneal Surgeries

Now that the overall context of possible ailments of the cornea and neighboring tissues has been explored, we turn to the fascinating topic of corneal surgeries, most of which have only recently been developed.

The cornea, as the clear portion of the eye, is most easily thought of as the windowpane of the eye. This pane can become damaged or diseased as we have seen, resulting in swelling, scarring, or other distortions which may reduce vision or even cause blindness.

To restore vision, the cornea may need to be replaced. This is referred to as a *corneal transplant* or a *penetrating keratoplasty* (Fig. 11-2). Corneal tissue is available from the local eye bank. The processing of a donor cornea goes through many control steps, assuring sterility from bacteria and other infectious agents such as hepatitis and the HIV virus. Once the cornea has been cleared, it is carefully stored and refrigerated until ready for transplantation.

In brief, the operation consists of transferring the central portion of the donor cornea to the patient's eye. Once this is done, the cornea is stitched to the patient's eye with many tiny sutures. The sutures typically are not easily seen with the naked eye and are not irritating. The length of time for a corneal transplant depends on the complexity of the disease process and the other procedures that need to be done such as cataract extraction, artificial lens implantation, or cleaning up the vitreous gel, usually from 45 minutes to several hours.

Soon after the operation, an eye patch and shield are placed over the patient's eye. The patient can walk about and resume normal routine activities while being careful to avoid bumping the eye. The return of vision depends on many factors, especially the individual's rate of healing and the health of the rest of the eye. Antibiotics and steroids are usually given after surgery to minimize infection, inflammation, and graft rejection. The eye should become more comfortable as each day passes. If there are any changes such as more redness, change in vision, or light sensitivity, it may be a sign of graft rejection. This can occur weeks to years after the original operation.

The success rate of simple corneal transplantation is excellent, approximately 95 percent success. Transplanting under conditions such as corneal degeneration from a cataract, corneal edema after cataract surgery, and in the treatment of keratoconus also typically have high success rates. Transplants for corneas that have had acid or alkaline chemical burns have lower success rates due to the extensive damage which usually characterizes such injuries.

It takes several days for the new epithelium to heal over the transplanted graft, during which the doctor keeps daily track of the process of healing. Then visits to the doctor may become less frequent and subsequent visits may be in one to two month intervals. Some sutures may need to be removed to improve vision and cause the cornea to return to a more normal shape. Contact lenses and glasses may be prescribed as the visual recovery process and healing are occurring.

Lamellar keratotomy (LK) is a form of cornea transplant that involves only the outermost layer of the cornea. The layer is removed and replaced with a clear non-diseased donor cornea. LK is used only to treat corneal diseases that result in darkenings which are slight and limited to the superficial layers of the cornea, such as in cases of injury scars, Reis-Buckler's dystrophy, Salzmann's nodular dystrophy, and spheroid degeneration. Selection of a patient donor and post-operative care are similar to that for a complete corneal transplant.

The presence of a chronic infection, degenerative processes, or injury to the cornea may lead to thinning and subsequent perforation of the cornea. A perforated cornea makes the eye and its contents readily susceptible to secondary infections, and of course the hole permits leakage of fluid. To prevent this, the hole in the cornea can be covered with a glue such as cyanoacrylate adhesive, a simple procedure performed in the doctor's office. This glue temporarily covers the hole in the cornea giving the cornea time to heal over the hole. It also allows time for corneal transplant surgery to be scheduled if necessary.

Modern technology and advances in surgical and antibiotic treatments have made confronting and resolving problems infinitely easier than was the case only a short time ago. In most cases, the important matter is to spot what is going on early enough so that a rapid treatment can begin. The importance of recognizing that your symptoms need treatment is strongly emphasized.

Wrap-Up

- Whenever possible, use "hypoallergenic" or allergy-tested eye make-up products.

- Discard wet make-up, such as mascara, if your eye becomes infected. Replace with new sterile products once the eye is healed.

- Keratoconjunctivitis sicca (KCS) or Sjogren's syndrome is the most common eye problem associated with rheumatoid arthritis (RA). Symptoms include red eyes, dry eyes, light sensitive eyes, and a sandy sensation in the eyes. KCS is present in 15.25 percent of RA patients.

- Acid burns tend to coagulate epithelial and stromal proteins, forming a material barrier or deep penetration into the eye.

- Alkaline absorbs into and penetrates the cornea and may inflame or damage the front half of the eye.
- Infections of the eyelids are very common. Prevention includes abstinence from rubbing your eyes, use of deodorant soaps when possible, avoidance and/or treatment of allergies, and the use of hot compresses when symptoms first appear.
- Any gray area on your cornea associated with pain, light sensitivity, "red eye," and decreased vision should be evaluated and treated by your ophthalmologist immediately.
- Adequate treatment of eyelid infections may take a number of months.
- The use of eyeglasses with UV 400 coating to protect you from ultraviolet light is especially important if you appear to be developing pinguecula or pterygium.
- The use of hot compresses, artificial tears, especially preservative-free tears, and an ophthalmic lubricant ointment at bedtime help relieve your dry eye symptoms.
- Subconjunctival hemorrhages look terrible and usually enlarge within the first three days. They require approximately one month to disappear. The treatment involves the use of ice compresses for three days followed by hot compresses until resolved. They are not threatening to your vision.

DRUG	SIDE EFFECTS
Bacitracin™ (Bacitracin Zinc)	Local irritation, stinging, burning
Bleph-10™ (Sulfacetamide Na)	Local irritation, stinging, burning
Blephamide™ (Sulfacetamide Na/Prednisolone Act.)	Elevated IOP, cataract, delayed wound healing
Chlormycetin™ (Chloramphenicol)	Bone marrow hyperplasia, aplastic anemia
Ciloxin™ (Ciprofloxacin HCl)	No definitive studies currently
Dexacidin™ (Neomycin, Polymyxin B Sulfates, Dexamethasone)	Elevated IOP, cataract, delayed wound healing
Garamicin™ (Gentamycin Sulfate)	Nephrotoxicity, neurotoxicity, fetal damage
Ganstrin™ (Sulfisoxazole Dipolamine)	Local irritation, chemosis, itching
Maxitrol™ (Neomycin & Polymyxin B Sulfates, Dexamethasone)	Elevated IOP, cataract, delayed wound healing
Neosporin™ (Polymyxin B Sulfate, Neomyxin Sulfate, Gramcidin)	Itching, conjunctival injection, edema
Polysporin™ (Polymyxin B, Bacitracin)	Hypersensitivity reactions, delayed wound healing
Polytrim™ (Polymyxin B, Trimethoprim Sulfate)	Local itching, burning, redness, stinging
Sodium Sulamyd™ (Sulfacetamide Sodium)	Local irritation, stinging, burning
Tobrex™ (Tobramycin)	Lid itching, swelling, redness, localized toxocity
Tobradex™ (Tobramycin, Dexamethasone)	Lid itching, swelling, redness, localized toxicity, increased IOP, optic nerve damage, cataract

Table 11–1 List of frequently used antibiotic medications.

Chapter Twelve

Buying Glasses

Consumer Reports, August 1993

Not that long ago, buying eyeglasses was about as simple and as uneventful as buying orthopedic shoes. Optometrists sold most pairs, usually basic spectacles in serviceable if unlovely frames, after an eye exam revealed the need for corrected vision.

Some time between then and now, these modest medical devices became fashion items, the profit center of a considerable retail industry. Eyeglasses from designers like Armani cost $200 or more—for the frames alone. A pair of lenses can add well over $100 to that, depending on the material, the optical specifications, and special coatings. Throw in the cost of an eye exam, and a pair of spectacles can cost as much as a modest color TV set.

The eyeglass business has become big enough to attract some of the country's corporate giants. The company that owns *Pearle Vision* is also parent to Burger King. *LensCrafters, Pearle's* arch rival, was the brainchild of former Procter & Gamble marketing executives; it is now owned by U.S. Shoe. Together, these two chains—the country's biggest—run more than 1,500 optical stores and cover most states. They have invested heavily in "superstores"—eyeglass emporiums where consumers can have their eyes tested, choose from thousands of frames, and, for many prescriptions, have glasses made in an in-store laboratory within about an hour. Smaller chains like

EyeMasters, For Eyes, and *Sterling Optical* have expanded to compete with the big ones.

To find out how well these chains served our readers, and whether they are better or worse than more traditional ways of buying glasses, we surveyed some 71,000 CONSUMER REPORTS subscribers who had bought prescription glasses in the previous two years—some at a private office, some at independent optical stores, and some at a big chain. We asked readers to tell us how satisfied they were overall with their experience of buying glasses, and asked some specific questions about cost, service, and other factors. Among the results:

Independent opticians and private optometrists and ophthalmologists who sell glasses as a sideline generally pleased readers more than did the big optical chains. They also offered glasses at prices that were competitive with the large chains.

Almost half the readers who bought glasses at one of the big optical chains complained that they'd paid more than they expected to. About one reader in six spent $250 or more on a pair of glasses. But some chains were far less expensive than others: The average price for a complete pair of glasses ranged from $88 at *Frame-n-Lens* to $192 at *Eye Masters.*

The readers who were most satisfied were generally those who bought from the chains that charged the least.

Almost half of those who bought glasses from a big chain had to return at least once because of a problem with the spectacles—often because the frames needed adjusting, and occasionally because a lens had come loose.

Readers examined by private optometrists and ophthalmologists generally found the examination very thorough; those examined at optical chains were much less likely to feel they had had a very thorough exam.

Satisfying Customers

The great majority of respondents had worn glasses for years. Three-fourths said they wear glasses most or all of their waking hours; more than a third wear bifocals.

Many of the survey respondents who bought glasses from a private optometrist or ophthalmologist said they made that choice because they had dealt with the doctor before and liked the service they had received. But many of those who bought glasses at the big optical chains had been drawn there by advantages private practitioners can't offer: a choice of convenient locations, ample frame selection, speedy service and special discounts.

The large chains themselves were fairly well liked by the people they served, as our Ratings show. But satisfaction was higher with private practitioners, taken as a group, than with most of the chains our readers tried.

Examining the Examiners: What an 'Eye Doctor' Does

Opticians, optometrists, and ophthalmologists may all play a role in the process that leads from blurred newsprint to a pair of specs. Here are the differences among them and what they do.

Opticians are technicians who make and fit eyeglasses and, in some places, dispense contact lenses. They cannot write a prescription for corrective lenses or diagnose disease. Only about half the states require formal licensing for opticians; in the others, just about anyone can hang out a shingle. A poorly trained optician may have particular difficulty fitting complex glasses, such as bifocals or glasses with progressive lenses. A state license or certification by the American Board of Opticianry may be an indicator (but not a guarantee) of appropriate training.

Optometrists earn a doctor of optometry degree, the O.D., from a four-year college of optometry, which they usually attend after graduating from college. They learn how to examine eyes, diagnose eye disease, and prescribe glasses and contact lenses. Different states define the limits of their practice differently. Two-thirds of the states let O.D.s prescribe certain drugs to treat eye disease—antibiotic drops for eye infections, for example.

Ophthalmologists are medical doctors who have completed several years of residency studying, diagnosing, and treating eye disease. Unlike optometrists, they can perform surgery. Some health maintenance organizations use ophthalmologists only for eye surgery or other treatment of eye disease or injury, reserving staff optometrists for routine eye exams. More and more, however, private ophthalmologists are checking eyes and selling eyeglasses and contact lenses.

About half the readers in our survey had their eyes examined by an optometrist, half by an ophthalmologist. The bulk of people who used a major eyeglass chain were examined by optometrists. Most people paid somewhere between $40 and $60 for an exam and felt it was thorough. A thorough exam should include the following:

- **History.** The examiner should take a record of past and current eye problems, systemic disease, and family history. Diabetes and high blood pressure in particular can damage blood vessels in the retina, causing serious vision problems or blindness. The examiner should ask about any particular visual demands from your job or hobbies and any medications you take.
- **Eye coordination.** This test tracks how well your eyes work together as you follow the doctor's finger or other target.
- **Visual acuity.** The doctor uses the familiar eye charts to gauge far and near vision, with and without glasses.
- **Eye structures.** A "slit lamp" plays light across the eye, allowing the examiner to check the lids, cornea, iris, pupil, and front of the lens. An "ophthalmoscope," a lighted magnifier, allows the doctor to see the back of the eye—the retina and part of the optic nerve. Sometimes, the pupil is first dilated with eye drops, to give a wider view.
- **Refraction.** A "phoropter," an apparatus you look through with dial-in lenses for all possible prescriptions, lets the doctor determine the amount of refraction—bending of light rays—needed to correct your vision to normal.
- **Intraocular pressure.** Some doctors use an air-puff machine to measure pressure inside the eye; high pressure is the cause of glaucoma. More precise measurement requires the use of drops to anesthetize the eye and an instrument that gently presses against the eyeball.

- **Field testing (peripheral vision).** The doctor will sometimes check your peripheral vision informally, bringing his or her fingers alongside your head and asking where you can or can't see them. Or the doctor may use a mechanized field test, one that uses small flashing lights. Measuring peripheral vision can uncover retinal damage, other eye disease, or neurological problems, including certain brain tumors.

The American Optometric Association recommends a yearly exam for everyone from preschool to age 25, exams every two years between ages 25 and 35, and annual exams again for those 35 or older. If you do not have eye problems, however, you can probably have your eyes tested less often. There are two important exceptions, noted by the U.S. Public Health Service: Diabetics should undergo an eye exam for possible retinal damage every year. And people at high risk for glaucoma—African-Americans over age 40 and all people over age 60—should be examined at least once every two years. In both cases, the Public Health Service says, the patient's pupils must be dilated by the doctor for a better view of the retina.

What Should Glasses Cost?

The top three chains in the Ratings—*Price Club Optical, For Eyes,* and *Frame-n-Lens*—are all distinguished by their emphasis on low prices. At *For Eyes* and *Frame-n-Lens,* most customers left with a pair of eyeglasses for less than $100, about 40 percent less than the average $164 charged at the big chains. (Glasses bought at private practitioners' offices averaged $158.) Readers who bought from the top three chains were significantly more satisfied with their experience than were readers who bought from more expensive stores. Glasses from *Price Club,* typically around $112 a pair, were especially valued for the high quality of their frames and their lenses.

High eyeglass prices reflect the fat markups on frames that are standard in the trade. The chains often charge double or triple the wholesale price, or more. (The average cost of $164 for a pair of glasses at the large chains includes $89 for the frame.) Frames with designer names are especially pricey. At a recent visit to a *LensCrafters* outlet in Manhattan, a CU reporter spotted a small, wire-rimmed Armani frame for $230. Opticians, we learned, buy the frame for just $68.

The president of *LensCrafters* says the high price of glasses reflects all the personal service involved—someone prepares and inserts lenses into frames and fits the glasses to the buyer. Yet some chains sell the same glasses far more cheaply than others, no doubt because they are more willing to settle for a lower markup than the 100 percent or more some add to the wholesale price of frames.

While the Ratings show which chains charged our readers most and which charged least, one can't predict which chain will have the best deal on glasses for a particular individual. We found that out when we sent three staffers—all nearsighted, one with a touch of presbyopia—to price glasses at New York-area branches of five major chains. Each staffer showed a prescription and asked for frames like those he or she was wearing; each requested the cheapest plastic lenses, then asked the price of anti-scratch coating.

The price differences between the most and least expensive chains were considerable: $176 versus $310 for one staffer, $142 versus $229 for the second, and $149 versus $195 for the third. *Sterling* was the least expensive chain in two cases out of three, and *Cohen's Fashion Optical* was the most expensive in two cases out of three. But one chain, *Pearle,* offered the cheapest glasses to one staffer and the most expensive to another.

Some chains are minefields of confusing—sometimes hidden— à la carte charges. At *LensCrafters* or *Pearle,* for example, you'll be quoted separate prices for the frame and for the lenses, with surcharges for add-ons like tints and coatings and for especially high-power lenses. (*Pearle* also charges extra for oversized lenses if a frame requires them.) Tints can be an especially big money-maker for the chains (the chemicals used to tint glasses cost only pennies). The Ratings show which chains tack on which surcharges.

One of the top-rated chains, *For Eyes,* offers not only low prices overall, but also a straightforward pricing policy: Prices are for complete eyeglasses, period, regardless of lens power or size. *For Eyes's* prices were among the lowest in our survey.

The pricier chains are also getting new competition from optical sections at discount and warehouse stores, the trade's latest wrinkle. These stores take a no-frills approach, offering a limited selection of frames in small facilities, sometimes just a corner of the store tucked behind the power-tools department or the grocery aisles. There may or may not be an optometrist on duty, and these places generally won't make glasses while you wait; instead, they send the order to an outside laboratory as private practitioners do. But the price might be worth the wait—warehouse stores cut their profit to the bone. (Warehouse stores often carry designer labels, too; a recent visitor to *Price Club* saw brands including Liz Claiborne, Polo by Ralph Lauren, and Evan Picone alongside cheaper, generic frames.)

Recently, *LensCrafters* and *Pearle* have also started going after the many folks who want to pay mass-merchandiser prices. *LensCrafters* is opening dozens of optical stores in K Marts under the name *Sight & Save* this year. There it will sell complete glasses at $39 to $99. And *Pearle* has installed an "Eye Buys" section in some of its stores: Complete glasses sell for $80, cheaper than many frames alone cost elsewhere in the same store.

Glasses to Go

Optical superstores with an on-premises lab can make most glasses in much less than a day (although some lens coatings and prescriptions, especially for bifocals, can take longer). In our survey, readers reported that the fastest chains were *EyeMasters, LensCrafters,* and *OptiWorld,* all of which managed to fill more than half of their orders in less than a day. *LensCrafters* ads promise to produce glasses within an hour, and 56 percent of the chain's customers in our survey said they received their glasses that quickly. In all, 83 percent said their glasses were ready by the day's end.

The longest waits were at *Price Club, Frame-n-Lens, For Eyes, Sears,* and *Royal Optical,* where most customers waited at least a week for their glasses. About one-quarter of the readers who went to Royal complained that the glasses weren't ready when promised. The same number complained that *EyeMasters* stores were too slow:

Although *EyeMasters* was faster than most other chains, it was not as fast as readers said they had been led to expect.

In principle, even stores without an on-premises lab may be able to get you glasses in a day or so on special request. *For Eyes* and *Sears,* for example, electronically transmit orders to a central lab. If you visit the store early enough in the day, overnight air delivery can return the finished spectacles the next day or the day after that. Both chains told us they don't charge for the service. *Frame-n-Lens* can put a similar rush on your order for $12 extra.

The Specs on Specs

How Glasses Fix What's Wrong

In normal vision, the eye's cornea (the clear outer layer) and its lens focus images on the retina at the back of the eye (see Figure 12–1).

Myopia (nearsightedness) results when incoming light from distant objects focuses in front of the retina, usually because the eyeball is elongated. Close vision is fine, but distance vision is poor. A concave lens, thinner at its center than at the edge, corrects the focus by moving it back onto the retina.

Hyperopia (farsightedness), less common than myopia, often results when the eyeball is too short; light rays are bent in a way that would focus on a point behind the retina. Distance vision is no problem; close vision is. A convex lens, thicker at the center than at the edge, corrects the focus by moving it forward.

Presbyopia is the common, gradual loss of the ability to focus on very close objects, caused by stiffening of the eye's internal lens after age 40. Reading glasses with lenses similar to those worn by farsighted people will help many people with presbyopia; bifocals or progressive lenses can help others.

Astigmatism is an irregularity of the cornea that blurs vision in one direction, an effect something like a funhouse mirror. Cylindrical lenses (shaped differently from the usual spherical lens) help compensate. The axis of the cylindrical lens must be oriented precisely so that it exactly cancels the distortion produced by the cornea.

Buying Glasses

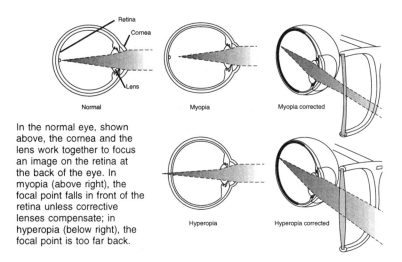

In the normal eye, shown above, the cornea and the lens work together to focus an image on the retina at the back of the eye. In myopia (above right), the focal point falls in front of the retina unless corrective lenses compensate; in hyperopia (below right), the focal point is too far back.

Figure 12–1

Turning 'Blanks' into Lenses

Opticians don't need to grind their own lenses any more. These days, stock lenses, called "blanks," are ground to different prescriptions by the manufacturer and shipped to the stores where they are sold. (For more complex prescriptions, the manufacturer will grind the front of the lens only, and leave it to the optician or optical laboratory to do the back surface. But the equipment required to do that is complex and expensive, and not all stores have it.)

With a little equipment and a couple of filing cabinets of lens stock, a small "finishing" lab in a store's back room can quickly trim a blank to fit a frame, a process called edging. Edging machines look and work something like the machines locksmiths use to copy keys: A template for a frame's eye shape guides a cutting arm that shapes the lens's outline.

This process, though automated, leaves room for human error. The blank and the template must be mounted precisely in the edger or else the lens's optical center won't be in the right place for the glasses. The lens must also be inserted into the frame precisely: With some prescriptions, an error of a few millimeters can result in visual problems for the wearer.

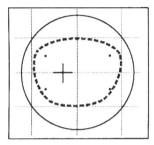

Figure 12–2   Edging trims a circular blank into a lens (broken line). Cross hair shows optic center.

Fitting a Frame

Our survey showed that more readers chose metal frames than plastic, despite the metal frames' often higher price. (The latest craze, titanium frames, can cost $200 or more.) But much more important than the material is the fit. The diagram below shows the fine points of fitting a frame to your face. Some general points to keep in mind:

- The lenses must be positioned properly—with their optical centers directly in front of the pupils—to prevent headaches and eyestrain. In positioning the lenses, the person fitting the glasses should take the asymmetry of the face into account; the nose is rarely centered exactly. Accurate positioning is especially important if you wear strong prescription lenses, bifocals, or "progressive" lenses (no-line bifocals).
- Avoid oversized frames, which require oversized lenses. Big lenses add weight, can distort vision, can catch glare, and may cost more than standard lenses. If you are nearsighted and choose oversized lenses, the edges of your glasses may be quite thick; smaller lenses would appear thinner.
- If you or your children play sports, get sports frames for that purpose. These frames, which resemble goggles, are stronger than "dress" frames; and, unlike dress frames, they have no hinges or bridge that can snap and injure eyes. It may not help much to buy impact-resistant lenses if the frames are easily broken; many eye injuries are caused when frames snap.

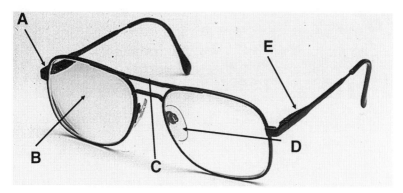

Figure 12–3 (A) **Hinges** Should be sturdy. Spring hinges, used on more expensive frames, help keep the eyeglasses from sliding down on your nose and stop the tendency for the sides to bow outward over time.
(B) **Eye shape** The size and shape should be appropriate for the face; lenses that are too big can look awkward and cause glare or distortion.
(C) **Bridges** Should not be too tight on the nose, but not too wobbly either. An extra crossbar here adds strength to the frame.
(D) **Nosepads** Soft silicone pads are comfortable and less likely than hard plastic to let glasses slide down when you sweat. Makeup will make silicone dirty, however. Hard pads on springs are another option.
(E) **Temples** The frame should not pinch or even touch the head until the point where it reaches the tops of the ears. The frame's sides should be long enough to bend down behind the ears to secure the glasses. To avoid obstructing peripheral vision—essential in driving and sports—the sides of the frame should be above or below the pupil of the eye, not level with it.

Bifocals—Three Different Ways

Bifocals have changed since Ben Franklin's day. They now come in three major styles, each with different advantages and disadvantages. The best type to use will depend on a person's needs and experience.

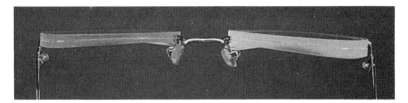

Figure 12–4A **Thick and thin** High-index plastics (right lens) are appreciably thinner and lighter than conventional lens material (left lens) in the same prescription strength. That can help the most-nearsighted people avoid glasses that would otherwise be extremely thick at the edges. Cost: $100 to $150, perhaps $25 more for oversized frames.

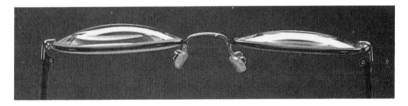

Figure 12–4B **Bulging and flat** Farsighted people must wear convex lenses (left lens), whose thick centers bulge outward and magnify the eyes. Aspheric lenses (right lens) have their front surface ground with complex and flatter curves for the same prescription; the wearer's eyes look more natural, too. Cost: $90 to $105.

Flat-top bifocals, the most widely used kind, have only a small area at the bottom for close-up work. The rest of the lens, used to see objects at a distance, offers good peripheral vision generally.

Franklin bifocals have the entire bottom half of the lens ground in the prescription for near vision. They offer the best wide-field vision for close work—ideal for accountants, graphic artists, and others who look at large sheets of paper.

Progressive lenses, the newest kind, are "no-line" glasses that gradually change lens power from top to bottom. They

Buying Glasses 199

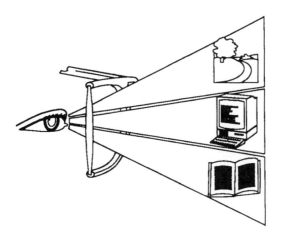

Figure 12-5 Progressive lenses are used for distance, mid-range, and close vision as the eye changes position.

give a continuous range of clear vision as eyes move from top (for distance) to bottom (for closest vision). Most important, the glasses offer a mid-range area—for viewing things at arm's-length distance—that is missing from regular bifocals, and that can be especially useful for people like musicians and computer operators. Progressive glasses take some getting used to—some wearers can never adjust—and the lenses, at about $150 a pair, cost twice as much as lenses for either kind of conventional bifocal.

Glassless Glasses: New Lenses, New Coatings

Glasses used to be made of glass. Plastic lenses are much more common these days; less than one-quarter of the readers in our survey bought spectacles with glass lenses. While glass resists scratching better than some plastic lenses, it's also heavy and more likely to shatter. The new kinds of plastic lenses, and the coatings offered with them, can pose some confusing choices.

Regular plastic lenses are made of a hard resin, called CR-39 in the trade; they weigh half as much as glass. These lenses should not need scratch protection unless the eyeglasses are likely to be handled roughly. They're the cheapest of the current options, at about the same price as glass lenses: $60 to $75 for a pair of regular lenses, more for bifocals.

High-index plastic lenses are at least 30 percent thinner than regular plastic lenses of the same prescription. This kind of plastic's refractive "index"—its ability to bend light—is so high that less of the plastic is needed. But these lenses are also expensive, costing $100 to $150 a pair, perhaps $25 more for oversized frames. The high price makes high-index lenses appropriate primarily for very nearsighted people, whose glasses would otherwise be extremely thick at the edges.

Polycarbonate lenses, almost as thin as high-index lenses, are made from a virtually unbreakable plastic that is also used in police visors and astronauts' masks. You can hammer polycarbonate and only nick it. Although polycarbonate lenses demand antiscratch coating—the material is softer than other kinds of plastic—they may be the best all-round choice. In particular, polycarbonate lenses offer a margin of safety for active people, such as children and athletes. They're even safer when the lenses are set in unbreakable sports frames, a crucial concern for avoiding eye injuries. At $80 to $95 a pair, plus about $20 for antiscratch coating, polycarbonate lenses cost somewhat more than regular plastic.

People who spend a lot of time outdoors in strong sunlight should be sure their lenses protect their eyes well from ultraviolet light, which can cause cataracts over many years. Glass filters out about 80 percent of UVB radiation, the kind associated with sunburn, but filters out very little UVA—a form of UV radiation that also appears to pose a potential health risk. Regular plastic filters out virtually all UVB rays and about 90 percent of UVA, while high index plastic and polycarbonate lenses filter out virtually all UV rays of both types. For extra protection, a UV-filtering dye can be added as a coating to regular plastic and glass lenses for about $20 to $25. Wraparound sunglasses offer even more protection, since ordinary frames allow sunlight in from the side.

People who are bothered by reflections in their glasses may also want to pay for an antireflection coating, similar to the coating on a camera lens. It costs about $40 or more.

Contacts vs. Glasses: Pros and Cons of Contact Lenses

For people who are always losing their glasses, who find frames chronically uncomfortable, or who simply can't stand the way they look in eyeglasses, contact lenses offer an alternative. In addition to their cosmetic benefits, contact lenses correct vision more effectively than eyeglasses; contacts move with the eyes, so the eyes always see through the lens's optical center. The result is crisp visual acuity, excellent depth perception, and natural peripheral vision. Contacts also never steam up, get rain-splattered, or smudge—and they don't bounce around your face or slip down your nose.

But contact lenses have their costs and risks. It's easy to spend hundreds of dollars a year on chemical cleaning systems for contact lenses. If you opt for disposable contacts to avoid the cleaning routine, the cost of weekly replacements can be even higher than the cost of cleaning.

Some kinds of contact lenses have been linked to eye infections and serious eye disease. The health risk stems from a basic problem of contact-lens design: The lenses need to sit atop the cornea, the clear outer layer of the eye, without choking off its oxygen supply. Oxygen-starved eyes are more vulnerable to disease.

The biggest problems have come from extended-wear lenses, which are designed to let enough oxygen through so that they can be worn continuously, day and night, for long periods. One theory is that wearing contacts at night when the eyes are closed may all but stifle the cornea's oxygen supply, despite the lenses' design.

Old-fashioned hard lenses, now used by only a tiny minority of those who wear contacts, were not designed to allow oxygen through; but they had to be removed often for comfort, and that let the cornea breathe. Soft lenses, now the most widely used type, are made of a plastic that lets some oxygen through during the day; more oxygen reaches the cornea when the lenses are removed every night.

A decade ago, some manufacturers promised that extended-wear lenses could safely be left in the eyes for a month. But recent studies have shown that these contacts and disposable lenses—essentially, extended-wear lenses meant to be thrown out after a week—can increase the risk of eye infections. One study found the incidence of ulcerative keratitis, a potentially blinding eye infection, was 14 times higher among people who used disposable lenses. Citing this and other research, the U.S. Food and Drug Administration has asked the makers of extended-wear lenses to recommend that they be worn for no more than seven days at a time. CU's medical consultants recommend taking extended-wear contacts out every night, or at least every other night—in other words, treating them more or less like regular soft lenses.

Given the problems with extended-wear and disposable lenses, it's not surprising that relatively few people use them; about five times as many people use conventional contact lenses that they take out and clean every night. While most of those people use soft lenses, many use what are called rigid gas-permeable lenses, made of a firmer kind of plastic. These lenses are somewhat more diffficult to adjust to than soft lenses, but they are easier to put into the eye and easier to care for, and they last longer. Soft lenses cost about $175 to $275 a pair for the original fitting (replacements are less); rigid gas-permeable lenses cost about $25 more. In contrast, extended-wear lenses cost $225 to $375 a pair, and disposable contacts cost $450 to $600 for a year's supply.

For people who decide contacts are too much trouble, going back to glasses is always an option. Eyeglass wearers outnumber contact-lens wearers by four or five to one, and the ratio isn't changing. One contact-lens specialist told us that for every person who begins using contacts, one user of contacts returns to glasses.

Decisions, Decisions

The process of buying glasses involves a series of choices. Should you go to a private office or a chain? Which lenses—and which extras—should you buy? Here's how the readers we surveyed made those decisions—and the probiems they faced despite their best efforts.

Chains vs. Doctors

Quality service and past dealings were the biggest factors that drew some readers to buy glasses from an ophthalmologist's or optometrist's private office. Those who patronized big chains most often cited convenient location and a good frame selection, along with speed and price—even though our survey showed that private practitioners often charge less.

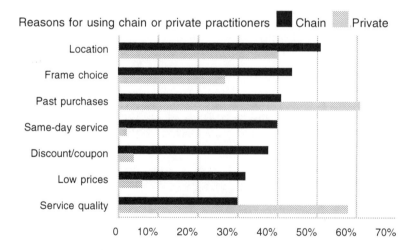

What They Bought

About three-quarters of readers bought just one pair of glasses at a time; another 23 percent got two pairs; 1 in 20 purchased three or more. Here's a rundown of the lenses and options they left with. (Percentages don't add to 100 because multiple glasses and multiple options may have been purchased.)

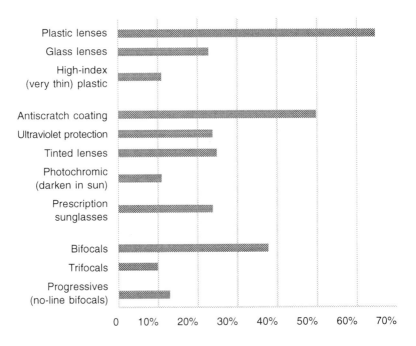

Eyeglass Problems

After wearing a pair of glasses for a while, about half the readers reported one or more problems. Most of those readers returned to the store or office with their glasses. Here are the percentages of all our respondents who reported each of the following problems.

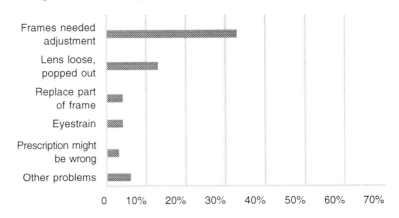

Personnel and Problems

Few stores stood out for their employees' attentiveness, courtesy, and knowledge. Workers at *Frame-n-Lens, Visionworks,* and *Opti-World* pleased readers most. At the opposite pole: *Empire Vision* and the lower-rated *Royal.*

While courtesy is nice, competence in a fitting is critical. About one-fifth of readers who shopped at the chains found their frames just didn't fit right. Additionally, some 4 to 8 percent of those who bought from the chains complained about each of these problems: glasses that caused headaches or other physical problems; lenses that were mounted incorrectly; or glasses with prescriptions that were not filled accurately. Half the survey respondents had glasses that often seemed fine at first but eventually developed problems. Most just needed a frame adjustment, but in one of eight pairs a lens came loose or popped out.

Overall, *Price Club* had the best record for selling problem-free glasses. *Royal* had the worst: Three-fifths of *Royal's* customers eventually had to make a return visit. As a group, the independent practitioners provided glasses that caused slightly fewer problems than glasses from the average large chain.

There are many ways to wind up with the wrong glasses. In some cases, the prescription is right but the lenses aren't inserted properly into the frames. In properly aligned glasses, the optical center is directly over the pupil of your eye. When alignment is off, the fault may lie with the lab or with whoever measured the eyes, sometimes a clerk using a ruler rather than a professional optician.

Positioning is especially important if you need strong corrective lenses or bifocals or progressive lenses—the "no-line" alternatives to conventional bifocals. In our survey, 19 percent of bifocal wearers complained that the bifocal line was too high or too low. The eyecare experts we spoke with stressed that anyone considering "progressive" lenses should be sure they can be returned or exchanged; many people find that those lenses are hard to adjust to.

You also need to buy lenses that will work well with your prescription and the kind of frames you're interested in. While regular plastic lenses are often adequate, polycarbonate lenses may be a better choice. Priced about $20 higher than regular plastic lenses, they are much thinner than regular lenses; they are extremely impact-resistant; and they filter out ultraviolet rays effectively.

Some stores may charge for polycarbonate lenses but insert the cheaper lenses. Last year, the New York attorney general claimed a *Cohen's* store in White Plains, N.Y., had "deliberately misled about the type of lenses" customers were getting. The store had been selling sports eyeglasses with regular plastic lenses, not the impact-resistant polycarbonate lenses that should have been used. In one instance, a boy's glasses shattered during a basketball game. The store admitted no wrongdoing but agreed to replace lenses in more than 100 pairs of glasses and to reimburse the state $20,000 in legal costs. (Another chain, *LensCrafters,* has just announced that it will use polycarbonate in all children's glasses at no extra charge.)

An experienced optician can tell what a lens is made of by noting its subtle coloration and tapping it with a fingernail. But ordinary eyeglasswearers can't tell the difference. Since there's no way to tell for sure whether a store is trustworthy, consumers must go by word of mouth.

By that yardstick, the *For Eyes* chain stood out in our survey—25 percent of readers who shopped there said the chain had been recommended by family or friends. The average chain got only 13 percent of its customers through such referrals. Further, *For Eyes* won more repeat business than any other chain: More than three-fifths of its customers had bought glasses there before and were satisfied enough with that experience to go back.

Ratings

Eyeglass stores

Listed in order of overall satisfaction with buying eyeglasses, based on responses to CU's 1992 Annual Questionnaire. Of 71,000 readers who had bought glasses in the previous two years, nearly 15,000 had bought from one of the chains rated below. Each chain was evaluated by at least 200 respondents. Results reflect the experience of our readers, not necessarily that of all eyeglass buyers.

1. **Overall score.** The average overall satisfaction with a chain, using the following scale: 100 = completely satisfied, 80 = very satisfied, 60 = fairly well satisfied, 40 = somewhat dissatisfied, 20 = very dissatisfied, 0 = completely dissatisfied. Differences of about three points or less between chains are not meaningful.
2. **Percent highly satisfied.** The percentage of survey respondents who said they were "very" or "completely" satisfied. Differences of 11 points are meaningful.
3. **Eyeglass price.** The median price readers reported having paid for a complete pair of eyeglasses. The margin of error for these estimates ranges from as little as $3 for the largest chains, *LensCrafters* and *Pearle,* to $10 or $15 for smaller chains. Note that different chains may sell a different mix of frame and lens options, which may account for some price differences.
4. **Extra charges.** Some chains say they routinely tack on charges for **oversized** lenses, **high-power** prescriptions, or **anti-scratch** coating. √ indicates an extra charge; — indicates the company include sthe option at no extra coast; V indicates charges vary among branches.
5. **Satisfaction with specific factors.** Readers told us how satisfied they were with different aspects of buying glasses: price, quality of frames and lenses, the speed of producing glasses, service, frame selection, and store hours. We have noted areas where satisfaction was higher or lower than the average for all chains.

Company	❶ Overall score (0-100)	❷ Percent highly satisfied	❸ Eyeglass price	❹ Extra charges Oversized	High-power	Antiscratch
Private offices[1]		71%	$158	V	V	V
Price Club Optical[2]		66	112	—	—	—
For Eyes		64	98	—	—	✔
Frame-n-Lens		64	88	—	—	✔
Visionworks		61	171	—	—	—
Opti-World		60	161	—	—	V
Vision World		57	96	—	—	✔
Eye World		53	158	—	✔	—
LensCrafters		55	182	—	✔	✔
Sterling Optical		51	137	V	V	V
NuVision		50	154	—	✔	✔
EyeMasters		48	192	✔	✔	✔
Empire Vision Center		49	113	V	V	√
Pearle Vision Center		48	173	✔	✔	✔
Cohen's Fashion Optical		47	187	✔	✔	V
Texas State Optical		47	175	—	—	✔
Sears Optical		47	166	—	—	✔
D.O.C Optical Centers		46	188	—	✔	✔
Royal Optical		40	146	V	✔	✔

[1] Average responses from 23,000 readers who bought from private optometrists or ophthalmologists.
[2] $25 annual membership fee required for warehouse store.

Location	❺ Satisfaction with specific factors
All states	Much higher satisfaction with service; higher satisfaction with price and quality.
Ariz., Calif., Colo., Conn., Md., N.J., N.M., N.Y., Pa., Tex., Va.	Much higher satisfaction with price, and higher satisfaction with quality—but lower satisfaction with speed of producing glasses and store hours.
Calif., Fla., Ga., Ill., Mass., Md., N.J., Pa., Va.; Wash., D.C.	Much higher satisfaction with price, but lower satisfaction with speed of producing glasses.
Calif.	Much higher satisfaction with price, and higher satisfaction with service.
Fla., Md., N.C., S.C., Va.	Much higher satisfaction with speed of producing glasses and frame selection; higher satisfaction with quality, service, and store hours.
Ala., Fla., Ga., Minn., N.C., S.C.	Much higher satisfaction with speed of producing glasses; higher satisfaction with quality, service, and store hours.
Conn., Fla., N.Y., N.J., Va.	Much higher satisfaction with price.
Mass., N.H., N.Y., R.I.	Higher satisfaction with speed of producing glasses and frame selection.
Most states	Higher satisfaction with speed of producing glasses; higher satisfaction with frame selection and store hours.
Calif., Colo., Conn., Del., Fla., Ill., Ind., Iowa, Me., Md., Mass., Mo., N.H., N.J., N.Y., Pa., Va., W.Va.; Wash., D.C.; Wisc.	Average satisfaction with all factors.
Ind., Mich., N.J.	Average satisfaction with all factors.
Ala., Ariz., Fla., Idaho, Iowa, Kan., La., Mo., Neb., N.M., Okla., Tenn., Tex., Wash.	Higher satisfaction with speed of producing glasses, frame selection, and store hours; lower satisfaction with price.
N.Y.	Higher satisfaction with price; lower satisfaction with service and store hours.
Most states	Lower satisfaction with price.
Conn., Fla., Mass., N.J., N.Y.	Lower satisfaction with price.
Ark., La., Okla., Tex.	Lower satisfaction with price.
All states	Lower satisfaction with speed of producing glasses and store hours.
Fla., Md., Mich., Mo., Ohio, Wisc.	Lower satisfaction with price.
Ala., Ariz., Ark., Colo., Fla., Ga., Idaho, Ill., Ind., Iowa, Kan., Ky., La., Md., Mich., Miss., Mo., N.M., Ohio, Okla., Ore., Pa., Tenn., Tex., Utah, Va., W.Va., Wyo.	Much lower satisfaction with speed of producing glasses; lower satisfaction with quality, service, and frame selection.

Recommendations

The most important step in buying glasses is the eye exam. While the big chains offer one-stop shopping with an eye test, there are advantages to having your eyes checked by an optometrist or ophthalmologist not connected with any store.

Our readers believed that private practitioners generally gave more thorough exams than those working in chain stores. In addition, private doctors are more likely to be objective about any problem you may encounter with glasses bought elsewhere. And a private doctor with no ties to an optician has no incentive to find that you *need* new glasses.

For people who want the convenience or large selection of a chain store, three chains offer good prices and were especially well liked by our readers: *For Eyes, Frame-n-Lens* and *Price Club Optical*. All three chains offered glasses at prices that were among the lowest in our survey.

None of those chains typically made glasses in a day, however, let alone an hour. If you're in a hurry, the quickest chains in our survey were *EyeMasters, LensCrafters* and *Opti-World*. All were significantly more expensive than the top-rated chains, however.

The best option may be to ask a store from a top-rated chain if your order can be rushed. Some stores will rush an order for an extra fee and some others will do so at no charge.

Wherever you buy your glasses, don't leave the store until you're sure you're happy with them. While progressive lenses often take some getting used to, ordinary new glasses shouldn't make you feel as if your height has changed or as if you're looking out from inside a fishbowl. If your glasses seem to distort your vision, either when you first buy them or later on, they may not have been made correctly. Discuss any problems you discover in the store right away, and don't hesitate to return to the store at any time in the future if you find that the glasses need adjusting.

Cheapest Chains

Median price paid for a complete pair of eyeglasses:

Frame-n-Lens	$ 88
Vision World	$ 96
For Eyes	$ 98
Price Club Optical	$112
Empire Vision Center	$113

Fastest Chains

Percent of customers whose glasses were ready the same day.

LensCrafters	83%
EyeMasters	68%
Opti-World	59%
Visionworks	49%
Eye World	46%

Best frame selection

Percent of customers who called the selection 'very large.'

Visionworks	64%
LensCrafters	52%
EyeMasters	47%
Eye World	46%
Opti-World	46%

Most Recent Business

Percent of customers who had bought glasses at the chain before.

For Eyes	62%
Sterling Optical	60%
Texas State Optical	57%
Vision World	52%
Frame-n-Lens	50%

Chapter Thirteen

Contact Lenses and Their Uses

Jim Pietrantonio

Basic Understanding

A contact lens is a small, dome-shaped transparent wafer worn directly on the eye's surface. Made of plastic or some other transparent material, it sits upon the eye's cornea or sclera, or in some instances both surfaces, hence the name.

A contact lens stays in place on the eye because of surface tension between the lens, moisture on the eye, and the eye itself, a phenomenon known to physics as "fluid attractional force." Just like a dime will stick to the tip of a wet finger, the contact lens will stick to your eye. The lens must be very close to the shape or contour of the eye surface to make surface tension possible. Most manufacturers make certain that the fit leaves a little steepness in the lens so that there is space between the center of the cornea and the contact lens. Tears fill this space with fluid, and coat the entire front surface of the contact lens (Fig. 13–1A and Fig. 13–1B).

Contact lenses don't sit rigidly in place. They tend to float downward during the first part of a blink, then back up to the origin as the upper lid is raised. This movement permits the nutrients in the tear film to be exchanged under the contact and keep the eye

Contact Lens Tear Layer

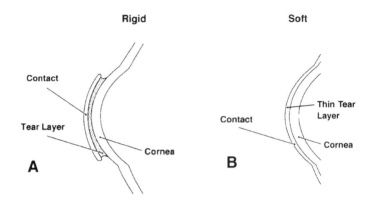

Figure 13–1 Contact lens tear layer beneath a soft and hard contact lens.
  (A) Hard contact lens with theoretical tear film present in between the cornea and the contact lens.
  (B) Large diameter soft contact lens with much thinner tear film.

coated. Too much lens movement may blur vision and irritate the eye. If this happens, the lens may need to be refitted. To avoid excessive movement, some contact lenses are fitted to the eye so that the upper eyelid covers a small portion of the lens. The lens is held against the cornea by direct pressure from the upper eyelid. Smaller lenses designed to adhere directly to the cornea can sometimes be caught by the eyelids and flipped out of the eye by an inexperienced user. This can occur if your eye has a significant amount of astigmatism.

Patients frequently ask, "Why do I see so much better with my contacts than I did with my glasses?" There are several reasons.

If you are nearsighted and put on your glasses, everything is in focus at distance, but is smaller than would be the case if you didn't have your glasses on. Compared with glasses, which are about one inch from your eye, contact lenses produce a relative increase in magnification simply because of the closer focal length to the cornea. Another aspect aiding improved vision is that with contacts, there is no longer any obstruction to vision made by a frame and the lens edge. Most important of all is that with contact lenses you look through the optical center of the lens and avoid the prismatic effect and peripheral distortions that are encountered when you look through the edges of your spectacle lens. This is especially important in prescriptions for higher correction levels. If you are farsighted, you may prefer the wider field of vision which contact lenses provide and not mind the slightly smaller image size you see. You certainly will not miss spectacles with their obtrusive weight and magnification and peripheral distortion factors.

There are several contact lens types, each with its own distinctive characteristics. The "corneal contact lens" is a lens whose diameter is equal to or less than the diameter of the cornea and which sits primarily on the corneal surface. Recently, rigid gas-permeable (RGP) lenses have been made of special plastics which allow oxygen to pass through the lens material, helping keep the cornea clear and pain free. While older lens materials cut off oxygen from the eye, limiting the duration of daily use, RGP lenses have almost unlimited wear time potentials. Most commonly, these are rigid contact lenses. Historically, rigid contact lenses were made of PMMA plexiglass.

A "water-loving" or "hydrophylic" *corneo-scleral contact lens*, generally referred to as a soft contact lens, is a lens that is larger than the corneal diameter and which covers both the cornea and a small portion of the sclera. This type of lens dominates the contact lens market at the moment.

Contact Lens Developments, Types, and Problems

Contact lenses go back a lot farther than most people think. The idea of an alternative to monocles or spectacles was first conceived two hundred years ago by lens grinders in Europe, and some lenses were actually made and tried out. These early contact lenses were crafted from ground and polished glass. They performed refraction adjustments moderately well, but they were large, heavy, and pretty uncomfortable. Since virtually no one could be persuaded to use them, the contact lens idea was set aside and stayed there until the mid-twentieth century.

By that time, lens-making technology had become a good deal more precise and delicate, and the physiological needs of eyes using contact lenses were more fully understood. In 1936, the Rohm and Haas Co. revealed its scleral contact lens made out of polymethylmethacrylate (PMMA), a plastic with the advantages of comparative lightness, acceptable precision in refraction, and a good deal less irritation to the eye than had been the case with the old blown glass contact lenses. For these reasons some wealthier patients at last began to accept the idea of contact lenses. PMMA plastic would dominate the contact lens market for most of the next four decades.

The big problem people had with using these contact lenses was that while they refracted radiation, the sections of the eye covered by lens were cut off from contact with the air. The hard PMMA lenses blocked adequate oxygenation of the tear film. When a cornea experiences a reduced oxygen environment, its center begins to swell and the surface epithelium develops fine water blisters in about one-half to three hours, depending upon the individual. When this happens, the swelling changes the cornea's curve which changes the refraction. Vision becomes blurred or fuzzy, the eye surface starts to hurt, and the eye becomes extremely light-sensitive. The solution is to take off the contact. Any widespread use of contacts would require inventing lenses with quite a high capacity for passing oxygen.

A partial solution was introduced in 1946, when Kevin Tuohy devised the smaller, lighter, and thinner corneal contact lens. It covered less surface area; therefore, patients could wear their lenses for longer periods of time and with considerably greater comfort.

Then in 1957 Otto Wichterle of Czechoslovakia developed the first soft, flexible hydrogel contact lens. It was made from a material whose lab name is hydroxyethylmethacrylate (HEMA). The Wichterle lenses were quite comfortable. Soft contact lenses can be bent or folded, yet when released return quickly to their normal shapes without damage. Hydrogel lenses have water caught inside and allow a reasonable degree of oxygen passage.

Low water content contact lenses are usually fitted as daily wear lenses and contain approximately 38 percent water. Low water content lenses generally have a correspondingly lower ability to pass oxygen through to the cornea. Low water content lenses should usually be taken out at bedtime or during any daytime naps longer than an hour or two, to prevent swelling from lack of oxygen.

Conversely, high water content lenses provide a much greater potential to deliver oxygen to the cornea. These lenses have a water content ranging from 55 percent to 79 percent and are thinner than low water content lenses. This design promotes the passage of oxygen to the cornea. High water content lenses are very comfortable, but they may be more difficult for you to insert or remove. Such lenses also are more fragile and easier to rip or tear.

At first, making hydrogel lenses was extremely time-consuming and therefore expensive, but in 1961 Wichterle invented a new, faster spin-cast method of fabricating hydrogel contact lenses, at which time their price per unit began to drop toward that of conventional eyewear. By the time Bausch & Lomb began its major promotion of hydrogel contact lenses in 1972, the pricing of conventional spectacles vs. contacts was nearly equivalent. The soft hydrogel lens has been further improved since then for better comfort and vision at a much lower cost. Today it is by far the most popular contact lens on the market.

In 1971, Norman Gaylord developed a rigid gas-permeable (RGP) material for contact lenses. Silicone methacrylate significantly improved the "breathability" characteristics of contact lenses and meant virtually an end to corneal edema, providing the patient took the lenses off at night to give the eyes a rest. Other RGP materials with even higher capacities for oxygen permeability, such as polyethylene, polystyrene, the fluorosilicones, and the fluoropolymers have been invented in the past quarter of a century, but they are much more expensive than silicone methacrylate and for that reason tend not to be the first choice for lenses recommended by eye care professionals.

Today the costs of producing lenses has declined to the point where even disposable contact lenses are available. It has been shown that lenses develop a coating of deposits in only a few days, which, while undetectable by the human eye, serve as a haven for microorganisms. This can produce either irritation or allergic reactions in the eye. Disposable contact lenses usually eliminate the need for lens deposit cleaning solutions (enzymatic cleansers). Since fewer contact lens care products are necessary, they also decrease problems with the eye's sensitivity to cleaning solutions.

Extended wear refers to the use of contact lenses on a continuous basis for 24 hours a day for several days. Usually the lenses are worn from two to seven days, depending upon the lens type and the individual patient.

The most common reason people give to justify wearing lenses without daily removals is that less cleaning and disinfection is needed. Also, removing lenses less often means less chance of losing or damaging them. The individual awakes in the morning and sees well immediately. The increased convenience is particularly important for those who travel on business, or who are maladroit with their hands.

All arguments in their favor aside, those who use extended wear contact lenses stand the greatest chance of experiencing problems with infection. Successful use demands your utmost attention to maintaining good wearing habits. Recent studies have indicated a 10-fold higher incidence of serious eye infections among extended wear patients. This can be substantially decreased if you are positively fastidious about using deodorant soaps on the face and hands. Many doctors now encourage all of their extended wear patients to remove their lenses as frequently as possible and to limit continuous wear of them to several days at a time. Most important, you should remove the lenses when you have a cold or flu, fever blisters, or any serious illness. You should inspect your eyes each day for redness. Any changes in the comfort of your lenses or in your vision, especially when a reduction of vision occurs in only one eye, could be a sign of trouble and reason to return to the eye clinic.

Tinted and colored soft contact lenses are slightly more expensive than clear lenses and are available in daily, extended, or as disposable wear lenses. A *tinted* soft contact lens is slightly colored to help in locating it either on or off the eye. This is particularly important if you have a high refractive error or are aphakic. The tint is so light as to have virtually no effect on your eye's appearance, and the light absorption is below that which would decrease light transmission. A *colored* contact lens has a "cosmetic" tint which changes or enhances the appearance of iris color. The greatest advantage of a colored soft contact lens, as opposed to a colored RGP lens, is that the center portion of the contact lens is clear so as not to dim light or change colors, unlike uniformly colored RGP contact lenses. The colored portion of the soft lens covers the entire iris, giving it a more natural cosmetic appearance. Colored soft contact lenses do not significantly alter color perception.

Cosmetic soft contact lenses are used to enhance iris color, but they can be quite valuable psychologically in instances of ocular disfigurement, albinism, aniridia (born without an iris), and other abnormalities. Colored soft contact lenses have the greatest enhancement effect on eyes with lighter iris colors. If a colored lens with the same color as the patient's iris is used, it results in a deepened tone. The cosmetic effect for darker irises is usually not as noticeable. The final effect on an eye is never completely predictable, and the only certain method of seeing the final outcome is to try them. Tinted or colored soft lenses may fade with time of lens wear, and the problem may be accelerated by the use of hydrogen peroxide disinfection systems to clean them.

Contact Lenses and Children

As a general rule, infants and young children are not fitted with soft contact lenses simply as a cosmetic substitute for spectacles. Getting these youngsters to properly take care of delicate lenses is problematic at best. If the need for soft contact lenses is not urgent, it is probably best to delay the fitting until the child is at least 10 to 12 years old.

On the other hand, contacts are suggested whenever they would be of advantage in assisting the development of normal binocular vision in a child. They can be helpful for infants and children with aphakia, certain types of strabismus (eyes are crossed or uncrossed abnormally), and the refractive type of anisometropia which could lead to a "lazy eye."

If children can see well out of both eyes, but have a big difference in the visual characteristics of each eye, contact lenses will significantly reduce the apparent difference between the two eyes. As a result, the youngster will continue to develop good binocularity as the eyes continue to grow. In amblyopic, lazy-eyed children, contacts sometimes are used as an alternative to covering the good eye with an "optical patch" as a form of therapy. A contact lens that is near focused is fitted to the good eye, and a distance contact lens (if needed) is fit to the "lazy eye." The amblyopic eye is then forced into use for distance viewing at all times. This works well and eliminates the inconvenience associated with patching, for example, removing and replacing the patch during the week. Most important, this technique also has the advantage of saving the child embarrassment. The contact lens therapy regimen works quite well as long as the contact lens stays in place on the eye.

Contacts and Astigmatism

Toric contact lenses are needed by patients who have astigmatism, either internal—the lens inside the eye is tilted—or external, as when the cornea is shaped like a football instead of like a basketball. To correct this astigmatism, you need a contact lens with two different power curves to neutralize the astigmatism. A lens with toric surfaces must be designed to orient properly on the eye and stay there within small tolerance limits. Toric contact lenses are more expensive because the fitting of the lens to the eye is more time-consuming, and usually each lens is custom-made for the unique prescription and shape of the eye.

Contacts and Presbyopia

Fitting older patients developing presbyopia, when the eye's lens loses elasticity and focusing on near objects becomes difficult, is the greatest challenge for anyone fitting contact lenses. This is because treating presbyopic conditions involves tinkering with a number of approaches, only some of which involve bifocal or other multifocal contact lenses.

An important consideration in fitting the beginning presbyope is the effect that the fitting of contact lenses will have on the refractive correction needed for near vision. This means if you are nearsighted and fitted for contact lenses in both eyes for distance, you will need reading glasses or bifocals for near work. Conversely, if you are farsighted and you wear contact lenses, your distance vision will be good, most of your intermediate vision will be good, and some of your near vision will be good. If properly fitted, slightly farsighted individuals generally do not need readers when wearing contact lenses.

Naturally, a successful *bifocal contact lens* fitting represents the ideal form of correction for presbyopic patients. However, the bifocal contact lens requires perfect fitting and even then may be insufficient for success. Another approach, referred to as *monovision contact lens correction*, involves prescribing single vision contact lenses by correcting one eye for distance vision and the other eye for near vision. Approximately 75 percent of such patients are able to adapt to the situation and function reasonably well. The correction for distance is usually awarded to the dominant eye.

Readers worn in addition to the contact lenses make close sight effective. But the most commonly successful remedy is for eye doctors to fit presbyopic patients with contacts that adjust refraction at a distance, providing readers or bifocals for close sight. This produces the fewest problems and complaints.

Bandage Soft Contact Lens

A *bandage soft contact lens* (BSCL) is any contact lens that is designed specifically for therapeutic purposes. These lenses are designed to transmit maximum oxygen to the cornea and to interfere as little as possible with normal corneal metabolism. The lens covers the entire cornea, and may or may not have corrective refractive power.

BSCLs are widely used to help patients with a variety of corneal abnormalities. For example, in *recurrent epithelial corneal erosion* there is a portion of the surface area of the cornea that never quite heals properly, usually after some sort of injury such as a scratch from a fingernail. Putting a transparent lens in place keeps air away from the fragile epithelial cells and cuts back loss of fluid through evaporation. The contact lens also protects the cells from the recurrent injury, such as the lid rubbing against the eroded area of the cornea. A BSCL is useful when eyelashes or lid sutures rub against the cornea, as in *trichiasis*. The eyelashes rub against the contact lens and not the sensitive cornea.

Another frequent use of BSCLs comes after eye surgery, for protection from sutures. Some eye surgeries require sewing very small stitches in the cornea, which can come in contact with the eyelid. Patients often feel the suture as the eyelid rubs across the eye during blinking or other eye movements. The BSCL eliminates this sensation until the sutures either dissolve, are covered with new epithelial cells, or are removed by the surgeon.

The BSCL can also be beneficial for some dry eyes because it protects the cornea from evaporation and holds a thin layer of tears against the cornea. BSCL therapy for dry eyes is more successful if artificial tears are instilled in each eye several times per day by the patient and the punctum of the eyelids have been closed.

Prosthetic Lenses

After a corneal injury or recovery from some other problem, an eye may have a different appearance. Contact lenses that are designed and fitted to the exact color and appearance of your eyes are termed *prosthetic lenses*. Today's soft prosthetic lenses are made from specially designed soft lens materials, or more commonly, thick molded "shells" custom made to fit your eye. The lenses are given a surface design with artificial coloring. The color and unique look of the iris can be determined from photographs, or through the use of trial lenses.

Contact Lens Fitting and Adaptation

The cornea depends partly on tears to supply nutrient materials and carry away metabolic waste. Stagnation of the tears under a contact lens can cause discomfort, redness, and even injury to the cornea. While the theoretical best case for fitting of RGP contact lenses is for the lens to float on the layer of tears and not to touch the eye at all, at least part of the lens does touch the cornea at all times. Understanding this, all attempts are made to limit the corneal touch, and to spread the lens pressure evenly around so that no localized abrasion or soreness occurs. The lens should fit the corneal contour closely enough so that lens weight is distributed evenly over a large area.

It usually takes about one to two weeks before anyone can wear RGP contact lenses for long periods of time, and about two to four weeks are required before the physiological adaptation is complete. Most people fully adapt to their contact lenses in a two-month period. Of course, adaptation time may vary for different individuals and different fitting techniques. The adaptation time seems to be faster for soft hydrogel wearers than for rigid lens wearers. If the new user experiences light sensitivity, prolonged eye irritation, red eyes, and blurry vision, the situation should be monitored immediately by the eye doctor.

While RPG contact lenses can protect the cornea from minor injuries, even chemical splashes, they offer no protection against direct hard impacts. The great majority of serious problems associated with contact lens wear come from patients' own poor attention to proper lens care and personal hygiene, particularly forgetting about arranging for follow-up examinations every three to six months.

The soft contact lens wearer usually has little or no adaptation problems, and this sometimes leads new users to think that follow-up examinations are not really necessary. That's pushing your luck. After the initial lenses have been dispensed, the patient should be allowed to build wearing time to achieve maximum daytime wear of 14 to 18 hours. Apparent adaptation is usually successfully completed during the first week after dispensing the lenses. Several follow-up visits are necessary initially, then one every six months.

As we have already seen, soft lens use dominates the contact lens market today. This user preference is due to several factors. Soft contacts are less likely to pop out from the eye's surface unexpectedly, or to dislocate from the cornea. Dust and foreign bodies usually do not get under the lens very easily. User adaptation time is significantly less than that required for RGP lenses, most soft lenses are easier and less expensive to fit, and soft lenses have both cosmetic and therapeutic values.

However, soft lenses are not without their disadvantages. Sometimes soft lenses don't provide good or stable vision. They are fairly delicate and can tear or split, and in fact don't wear or last as long as hard lenses. Perhaps the most significant downside of soft lens use is that wearers have more problems with infections. Soft contact lens solutions present a more complex problem for adequate disinfection and storage than do RGP lens solutions. There is also a greater opportunity for error, as some solutions may only be used with certain types of soft contact lenses. It is easy to get confused, so users should never change solutions without the approval of their doctor.

There are several types of solutions used in soft contact lens care. Wetting solutions are primarily used for rinsing or rehydrating lenses after insertion. Cleaning solutions are used to clean off deposits and contaminants. Disinfecting solutions are used against bacteria and viruses, and are applied in the contact lens case and before insertion. Enzymatic cleaners are effective in removing deeply bound proteins found beneath the surface of a soft lens. Finally, rewetting solutions are designed for use as eyedrops while the lenses are being worn, to lubricate and rehydrate them and make them more comfortable on the eye.

Infections and Complications

The biggest problem in keeping soft contact lenses clean is a very human one: denial. Many users fail to stick with the very procedures which protect them from infections, either because of asserted confusion about the procedures or because the procedures are too involved or time-consuming. Even when patients follow proper care techniques, periodic microbial contamination of the contact lenses or contact lens care systems is possible, simply because microbes are always around us, awaiting any opportunity to present themselves.

When infections occur, there is also a tendency in some people to procrastinate about having a doctor look things over. The patient hopes matters will clear up on their own account, saving the hassle of visiting a clinic. This can produce a gap in care which can be serious. Typically, cases of permanent eye damage among contact lens users come after the user fell into a pattern of negligence and improper hygiene. The most common causes of infection are unclean hands and skin, unclean contact lenses, contaminated solutions, local infections resulting from a corneal abrasion, or corneal foreign bodies. Most abrasions come from fingernails during insertion or removal, from foreign bodies pinned under the contact, or from general mishandling of the lens. If infection or ulceration is being treated, contact lens wear must be interrupted for a period of up to several weeks, depending on the severity of the infection or ulceration. It is possible to lose an eye, even with the very best of care and medications, if the organism is virulent and drug resistant.

Corneal ulceration represents the most serious complication to the cornea associated with contact lens use. It is not uncommon to find permanent scarring that is a direct result of contact lens wear. When scarring occurs, it is usually the result of an infection or improper wearing procedures. Scarring seldom occurs unless the patient continues to wear the lens, even though experiencing pain and light sensitivity.

Soft contact lens wearers occasionally develop tiny peripheral blood vessels growing into the cornea. In most cases, this *corneal vascularization* is caused by an improperly fitted contact lens or complications arising from a corneal injury or infection.

Very often the vascularization came about after an improperly-fitted soft contact lens was stuck too tightly in place for too long against the cornea, disrupting tear circulation and interfering with normal corneal metabolic processes. This creates "corneal hypoxia," or deprivation of oxygen to the cornea. The growth of the tiny vessels can be interrupted immediately if the patient stops using contact lenses, and the corneal vascularization usually disappears in a few months. *Corneal* or *stromal infiltrates* are white, cloudy spots usually seen in the stromal layer of the cornea. They occur irregularly among contact lens wearers, with or without infections. The infiltrates are typically found near the limbal area, where the cornea and sclera meet, but may occur at any position as patches of a hazy gray color. The eye may become very red, irritated and painful, or

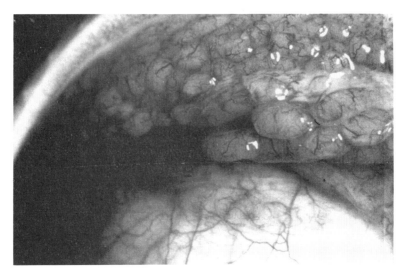

Figure 13–2 Everted upper eyelid revealing giant papillary conjunctivitis (GPC). GPC is usually associated with continuous soft contact lens wear, causing a large "cobblestone" formations on the inside surface of the upper eyelid.

may be "quiet" so that the patient may be totally unaware of any problems. Stromal infiltrates are often associated with chemical irritation from storage solutions, especially those including thimerosal. A hypersensitivity to staphylococcus organisms can cause a *staph marginal ulcer*. The contact lens should be removed until the infiltrate is no longer present and the source of irritation identified, if possible. Lens wear should not be resumed until the infiltrates have completely disappeared, which can take two to three weeks.

Giant Papillary Conjunctivitis (GPC) is often linked to contact lens wear, whether soft or RGP (Fig. 13–2). The symptoms of GPC include increased mucous secretion, itching, and increased awareness of the contact lens. Deposits from tears begin to accumulate on the lens surface and become denatured proteins. The re-formed lens proteins act as an antigen and stimulate an allergic response in the eye's tissues. The process is furthered by the effect of lids rubbing over the lens during the thousands of blinks that take place each day. Slowly and progressively, often over several months, the patient becomes completely intolerant of the contact lenses.

Alleviating GPC is difficult. Vigorous cleaning of the lenses is advisable but seldom solves the problem. Frequent lens replacement is more effective, but does not guarantee successful resolution. The only sure way to end GPC is to discontinue contact lens use until months or years have passed and the eye tissues have had the chance to "forget" about the allergic response.

Let me conclude this discussion by going over some of the more tangential uses to which contact lenses sometimes are now put.

Keratoconus and Corneal Transplants

Keratoconus is a noninflammatory, progressive corneal disease that in most cases affects the central portion of the cornea. It is characterized by a cone-shaped protrusion and thinning of the cornea. In its more advanced stages, keratoconus vision cannot be very well corrected by spectacles, but good results can be obtained through prescription of specially designed RGP contact lenses. If the cornea becomes excessively abnormal, it is replaced by normal tissue through corneal transplantation.

Contact lenses may also be recommended after a corneal transplant, if use will provide better vision than could be achieved with spectacle lenses. There are two major challenges involved: a visual problem and a physiological problem. Many transplants leave a patient with high refractive errors and/or irregular astigmatism in the corneal graft, possibly surrounded by a host cornea with different shape characteristics. Fortunately, in most cases a good optical result is achieved by wearing contact lenses (Fig. 13–3).

Orthokeratology

A curious use of contact lenses has been to reshape the corneal bulge. In "orthokeratology," RGP contact lenses are used in a deliberate attempt to flatten the cornea in the effort to reduce or eliminate nearsightedness. There are many variations in tech-

Effect of Tear Layer on Irregular Cornea

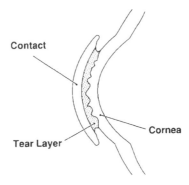

Figure 13–3   Schematic depicting how an optically perfect hard contact lens utilizes the corneal tear film layer to correct corneal irregularities.

nique, but the approach is usually to fit a patient with a series of RGP lenses over an extended period of time with each lens having a progressively flatter base curve. As the cornea flattens, the patient is fitted with new, even flatter contact lenses until the need for correction is eliminated. At that point, the wearing time is reduced gradually until at last the lenses are only worn part-time. Most studies indicate that orthokeratology patients with low refractive errors can have their vision improved through this means, but the process is expensive, its results are not permanent and it may produce a sense of chronic, moderate central corneal irritation.

Anisometropia

Patients with *anisometropia*, or large differences of refractive error between the eyes, usually benefit greatly from wearing contact lenses. Spectacle lenses present many problems for anisometropic patients. When they look through the center of the lenses, there is a definite, sometimes incompatible difference in image sizes. This effect increases when the two eyes are not directed toward the optical center of the lenses but sideways or downward. Either RGP or hydrogel contact lenses eliminate the problem because their refraction adjustment is on the eye's surface, not an inch away.

Are Contacts For You?

What goes into the decision to wear contacts? Some individuals make the choice on the grounds of better vision, others because they consider conventional eye glasses to be unattractive. Some choose to wear them, particularly the disposable contact lenses, because they seem more convenient. But not all patients can wear contact lenses successfully, and success rates depend to a degree on individual personality and proper follow up evaluations.

Perhaps the most important variables to consider if you are thinking about buying contact lenses are:

1. How much can you expect your vision to be improved with contact lenses as compared to your vision through eyeglasses?
2. Can you wear your contact lenses to work? If not, are evenings and weekends worth the costs?
3. How badly do you want to wear contact lenses?
4. What is your real motivation to wear contact lenses?
5. Do you have any systemic diseases or eyelid or corneal abnormalities which would prevent you from wearing contact lenses?
6. Do you have any diseases or conditions that would prevent you from inserting or removing your lenses, like rheumatoid arthritis or Parkinson's disease?
7. Are you ready to take on the regular cleaning and proper disinfection needed to prevent serious eye infections?

For any contact lens to be worn successfully, it must fulfill four basic requirements: it must correct your refractive problem, it must be comfortable, it must be physiologically compatible with the eye, and the desire to wear them must be decided. These requirements are fulfilled by choosing the proper contact lens type and dimensions. It may be necessary for the eye care practitioner to try out a number of different lenses with various diameters, base curves, and materials to assure you the best available comfort and vision.

Rarely does a new wearer feel discomfort or outright pain during fitting or wearing contacts, but the sensation of a foreign body on the eye may be uncomfortable during the trial wearing period. This may continue for several days. After this adjustment period, few wearers are much aware that they have contact lenses on their eyes.

Wrap Up

- Approximately 35 million individuals wear contact lenses in the United States.
- Approximately 23 million individuals attempt to wear contact lenses, but for one reason or another are unable to.
- Soft contact lenses are sometimes cheaper and more comfortable than semi-rigid gas permeable (RGP) lenses. However, your vision may not be as sharp with soft contact lenses.
- RGP lenses are easier to handle than soft contact lenses and do not need to be replaced as often as soft contact lenses.
- The wearing of extended wear soft contact lenses (one or more weeks at a time without removal) is not recommended. Currently, 95 percent of the complications associated with contact lenses are in extended wear users.
- Giant papillary conjunctivitis (GPC) is the most common significant complication of soft contact lens wear. GPC is relatively uncommon in rigid gas permeable contact lens wear.
- GPC's appearance is characterized by the presence inside the eyelids ranging from small bumps to large raspberry-like surface bumps. Increased mucus is also commonly associated with GPC.
- Preservative-free contact lens solutions are best to use whenever possible.

- Use only products that are part of your disinfecting system. "Mixing" and "matching" with whatever is on sale during a particular week may cause problems.

- Over 50 percent of contact lens cases are unsterile, so change your solutions and cases frequently. Ask your doctor.

- The use of deodorant soaps on the face and hands as often as can be tolerated by your skin is recommended.

- Wash your hands carefully before handling your contact lenses and your eyelids. This reduces the chance of infection and complications.

- If you are presbyopic (losing your ability to see up close), there are numerous fitting techniques and systems available.

- You do not have to worry about losing your lens and having it lodge behind your eye or around your brain. The conjunctiva covers the eyeball and the eyelid and is connected at the fornix thus preventing the contact lens from going behind your eye.

- There are important reasons why your contact lens doctor checks your eyes every four to six months. Keep your appointments.

- If your doctor has an economically planned contact lens replacement program, we suggest you use it. Frequent soft contact lens replacement helps prevent GPC, neovascularization (abnormal blood vessels) of the cornea, corneal ulcers, and other problems associated with contact lens wear.

Chapter Fourteen

Ophthalmic Plastic and Reconstructive Surgery

Martha C. Wilson

Ophthalmic plastic and reconstructive surgery works to improve and correct the function of tissues near the eye. Much of what is now possible has only become so because of rapid, dramatic improvements in knowledge, backed by a coincident growth in tested procedures and new technology.

A fundamental part of ophthalmic plastic surgery works to resolve circumstances which endanger the eye, or impede its functions. Until recently, plastic surgery appeared to be a realm in which the very wealthy toyed with Mother Nature and attempted to hold back the natural forces of aging for foolish reasons. Today, the psychological effects of cosmetic surgery are better understood. In a society which honors the physically attractive, tailoring of the external self has become accepted and nearly commonplace. It is possible to create an enhanced presentation to the world, and with good results.

Treatment of Function Problems and Disease

All of the conditions described below are considered medically necessary and treatment is payable by most insurance companies.

Most eyelid surgeries are performed on an out-patient basis. The surgery can be done in the hospital, in an ambulatory surgery center or, in some cases, in the physician's office when equipped with the necessary equipment. Usually an anesthesiologist provides intravenous sedation and monitors vital signs. While the operation is being performed under local anesthesia, the patient dozes. Therefore, he or she is comfortable and unaware of pain. During the operation, the patient is completely relaxed and "floating," but will be wide awake at the completion of the surgery.

The eyelids are the most important structures protecting the eye. They mantle the front of the eyeball and contour it tightly, leaving a relatively small aperture for vision. The eyelids are also responsible for keeping a thin film of tears on the surface of the eye. This film of tears is vital to the health of the cornea, and to permit rotation of the eye in its socket. Even small deviations from normal eyelid position can cause severe discomfort and can become an actual threat to vision.

Sometimes the upper eyelids weaken and droop low enough to partially cover the pupil and block some or all vision. This is called *eyelid ptosis* (Fig. 14–1A). Individuals with this condition are unable to see adequately; some actually need to lift the eyelid with a finger in order to see.

Drooping eyelids may be due to a child-related congenital defect that results from failure of eyelid muscles to develop properly. More frequently it occurs in adults and is caused by the stretching of any one of the muscles that lift the eyelid. Droopy eyelids can happen with age, or following eye surgery. Many times it occurs for no apparent reason.

There are nearly a dozen types of surgery for the correction of droopy eyelids, depending upon the exact cause of the droopiness. In general terms, most surgeries consist of "tucking," "shortening" or "lifting" muscles so that they can be stronger and pull the eyelid higher. Some patients require a reduction of the overhanging skin. Surgery can often be done from the inside of the eyelid, leaving no external scars. In other patients, the scar is hidden at the eyelid crease (Fig. 14–1B).

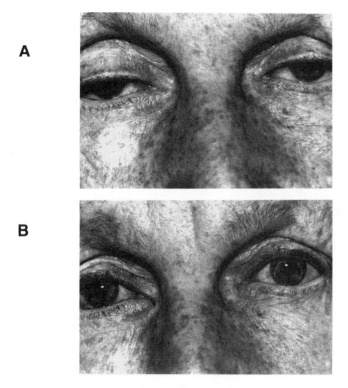

Figure 14–1 Eyelid ptosis before and after surgical correction.
(A) Before surgery, both eyes show extreme cases of ptosis, with eyelids partially blocking vision.
(B) After surgery, the eyelids are normal with vision unimpaired.

Droopy eyebrows, or *eyebrow ptosis,* occurs with age but may occur in younger individuals. When the droopiness of the eyebrows is to the point that they rest on the eyelids, rectifying the condition is considered medically necessary.

Baggy upper eyelids are ordinarily interpreted as a sign of age, but heredity can also produce this condition in young people. When the eyelids become so baggy that they partially block vision, they are considered to be a medical condition called *dermatochalasis*

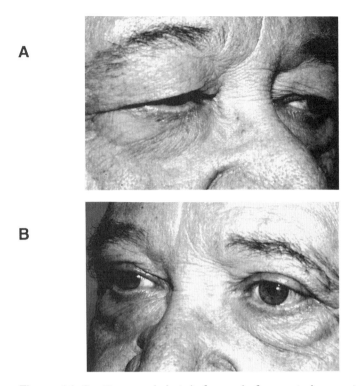

Figure 14–2 Dermatochalasis before and after surgical correction.
(A) Exhibits dermatochalasis with overhanging skin weighing heavily on the lashes.
(B) After surgery, dermatochalasis is corrected with the eyelid fold present.

(Fig. 14–2A). When baggy eyelids are left uncorrected, the overhanging skin weighs on the lashes. With time, the eyelashes become directed downward instead of upward. Eventually they may turn toward the eyeball, rubbing on the cornea. It is best to perform corrective surgery before this occurs because it is very difficult to turn the eyelashes out again. Surgery is an artistic matter of sculpting overhanging skin, muscle, and bulging fat (Fig. 14–2B). For this surgery to be considered "medically necessary" rather than cosmetic, the doctor must demonstrate that vision is impaired. A peripheral

Ophthalmic Plastic and Reconstructive Surgery

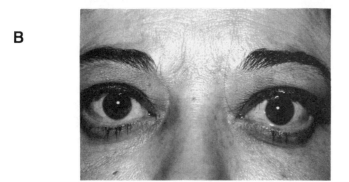

Figure 14–3 Eyelid retraction before and after surgical correction.
(A) Before surgery both eyes show an extreme case of eyelid retraction.
(B) After surgery, the condition is corrected, resulting in a normal appearance.

vision test and medical photographs are always used as evidence for the insurance companies.

"Staring eyelids" is where eyelids open too wide, producing a startlingly wide stare. The eyes in *eyelid retraction* are disconcerting to the onlooker; at best, the individual will look naive, but at worst the effect is of continual surprise (Fig. 14–3A). Eyelid retraction is found much more often in women's eyes than men's, and in fact from time to time it has been considered attractive, especially among *ingenues*. The most common cause of this condition is "thyroid eye disease," also called "Graves' disease." Tumors or inflammation behind the eye can also cause the eye to become more prominent. Eyelid retraction became the subject of intensive research in the 1980s after it was diagnosed in the former First Lady, Barbara Bush. Observant newscast viewers may recall how widely Mrs. Bush's eyes opened before she received treatment.

This condition underscores the importance of normal eyelid position for the health of the eyes. The big difficulty with eyelid retraction is that when the eyelid opening is abnormally large, higher evaporation of tears can produce dryness of the eyes. This is both uncomfortable and potentially dangerous, through higher likelihood of infection.

The appropriate surgery to cure eyelid retraction is to weaken the muscles that lift the upper eyelid (Fig. 14–3B). Because of the potential medical danger if surgery is not performed, the resolution of eyelid retraction is payable by insurance.

Looseness of the lower eyelid, or *lower eyelid laxity*, is usually associated with aging (Fig. 14–4A). The lax eyelid sags and is unable to adequately protect the eye, a situation producing continual tearing and the possibility of chronic eye irritation. The underlying problem is the stretching of the tendon that keeps the lower eyelid pulled snugly around the eye. Surgery is performed through a half-inch incision on the outer corner of the eye. The stretched tendon is removed and a new tendon is reconstructed out of stronger lower eyelid tissue. The new tendon is then fastened at the outer corner of the eyelid (Fig. 14–4B).

With a sagging lower eyelid, in-turning of the eyelid, or *entropion*, is common (Fig. 14–5A). This is a very uncomfortable condition because the lower eyelid's lashes and skin turn inward and rub against the eye, constantly irritating the eye and putting the eye at risk for infection or permanent scarring. The loose, unstable eyelid may suddenly "flip" inward, particularly during strong blinking. Sufferers of this condition typically find ways to ease their discomfort by keeping the eyelid from rolling in, but surgery is the only permanent solution (Fig. 14–5B).

The most successful surgical approach is to first treat the lower eyelid tendon, explained above. Then a horizontal incision is made

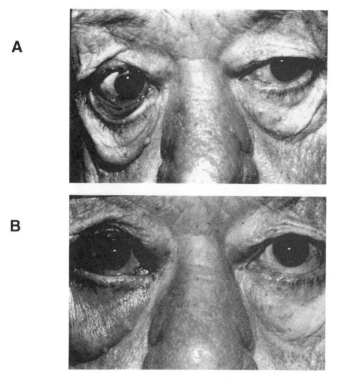

Figure 14–4   Lower eyelid laxity before and after surgical correction.
(A) This patient shows an extreme condition of lower eyelid laxity in which the lower eyelid will no longer protect the lowest portions of the eye.
(B) After surgery, the eyelid laxity is corrected, permitting improved comfort and health of the eye.

below the lower eyelid lashes. The lower eyelid muscles are then re-attached or cut away. The in-turned eyelashes are then rotated out with sutures. Most patients feel better immediately because the eyelashes are no longer rubbing against the cornea. Tenderness may last a couple of months.

Out-turning of the eyelid, or *ectropion,* is another uncomfortable eyelid condition. In this case, the lower eyelid is so loose that it falls outward, leaving the inside of the eyelid and part of the

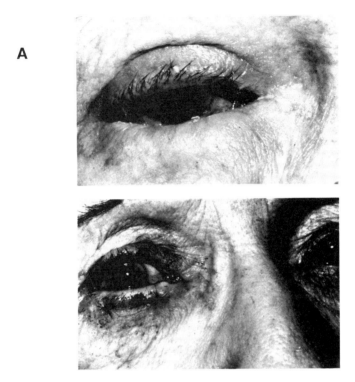

Figure 14–5 Entropion before and after surgical correction.
(A) Entropion with the eyelid and eyelashes rolled incorrectly against the cornea causing pain and irritation.
(B) This early post-operative period photograph shows the condition surgically corrected with the eyelashes directed outward.

eyeball exposed to the air. The result is a red, irritated eye. The surgical procedure for correction of ectropion is the same as for lower lid laxity.

Those who spend a great deal of time outdoors in sunlight increase their odds of developing cancers, including cancers of the eyelid. When a cancer occurs on the eyelid, it may be necessary to remove a section of the eyelid. If surgery is done when the tumor

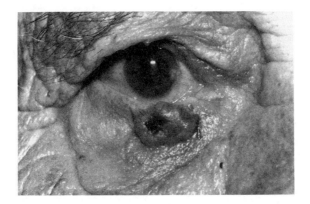

Figure 14-6 Basal cell carcinoma of lower eyelid.

is small, typically the eyelid can be put back together with specialized techniques. If the tumor is large, more of the eyelid must be removed and reconstruction can be difficult. For this reason alone, it is important to treat eyelid tumors as early as possible.

Basal cell carcinoma is the most common form of skin cancer of the eyelid, and for the rest of the body (Fig. 14-6). It usually does not spread to internal organs, but it may continue to grow and destroy local tissues. If left untreated, this cancer can grow into the eye socket and may result in total loss of the eye. The typical appearance of basal cell carcinomas are; rounded pearly margins, with central depressions, erosions, or ulcerations.

Squamous cell carcinoma is the second most common malignant tumor of the eyelids and surrounding areas. This condition is also associated with chronic sun exposure and is frequently found in middle-aged and older men. Squamous cell carcinoma is located on the lower eyelids, more often than on the upper eyelids. Tumors can spread in both locally invasive patterns and to regional lymph nodes. All suspicious lesions should be examined, biopsied, and surgically removed if possible.

Abnormal tearing, or tears running excessively down the side of the face, are uncomfortable and result in blurred vision. To understand why a person is tearing, one must first understand how tears are produced and drained out of the eye.

There are two types of tear-producing glands. The most important and largest tear gland is under the upper eyelid at the outside corner of the eye. There are also smaller glands located along the upper eyelid. Tears are swept across the eye by the action of the eyelids. Two small openings in the inside corners of the upper and lower eyelids drain tears out of the eye. These openings are commonly known as the tear ducts. The ducts are attached to very small passageways which empty into a sac on the side of the nose. From this sac, tears are drained out of the eye and into the nose.

When there is a blockage in the drainage system, tears will back up and run down the cheeks. Blockage of the tear duct system can occur after an infection, an injury, sinus disease, or result from other causes. A blockage can usually be spotted through an office procedure known as *lacrimal irrigation.* A small blunt needle is inserted into the tear duct and salty water is introduced. If no blockage exists, the patient will promptly taste the salty water.

Excessive tearing in babies or young children is frequently due to the blockage of a prenatal membrane that failed to dissolve after birth. Almost all infants with tearing can be treated merely with massage and medication. In the remainder of cases, the membrane can be "popped open" by inserting a thin wire into the duct. Older children may need tubes inserted into their tear ducts, and a very small number of these children require surgery.

If there is no blockage, yet the person still tears abnormally, the individual usually has one of two problems. These problems are: dry eyes, or flaccid lower eyelids.

Dry eyes are chronically irritated. This irritation leads to reflex production of tears which may not be "high quality" tears, that is, they may lack some of the normal components of tears. Tears produced naturally contain the lubricant mucin, and certain oily components as well as water. There are many causes of dry eyes, including natural aging. Dry eyes are treated with artificial tear drops. When used on a regular basis these drops help prevent irritation and thus decrease reflex tearing.

The other most common cause of tearing in adults is the obstruction of the tear duct system that occurs with age. A build-up of secretions in the tear sac located close to the inside corner of the eye may result in infection, causing a great deal of pain, abscess formation, and the need for strong antibiotics. Surgery is indicated not only to re-establish the drainage of tears but also to prevent infections. When performed early, surgery is effective in the majority of such cases. However, when this procedure is performed after an infection has already occurred, the success of the surgery decreases.

An eyeball may need to be removed because of trauma, tumors, or intense and persistent pain. Chronic pain and shrinkage of the eye can come about when disease has caused the loss of all useful vision. The small, blind, and painful eye can be removed and replaced by an artificial eye with great relief to the patient. Today it is possible to achieve a very natural appearance with an artificial eye. In many cases only the inside of the living eye need be removed, leaving the white shell intact.

When an eye is removed a "ball implant" is placed in the eye socket, covered with the same tissues that normally protect the eye. A custom-made artificial eye, or *prosthesis,* is then placed in front of the "ball implant" in a like manner to the way a contact lens is applied. The artificial eye, in fact, is like a large contact lens painted to resemble the healthy eye.

The bones surrounding the eye are very delicate, and even a relatively minor impact can result in fractures. Treatment of the broken bone material may require surgery where the broken bone is replaced by a plastic shelf or a bone graft. The best solution is not to endanger the bone in the first place.

Cosmetic Surgery

People first notice the eyes when they look at another person's face, and the contour of the eyelids is the most important factor determining how the eyes look. Depending upon their shape, the eyes can seem old, tired, or bored—or they can look rested, youthful, and energetic. So it is no surprise that cosmetic surgery of the eyelids constitutes much of the practice of the ophthalmic plastic surgeon. Cosmetic eyelid surgery seeks to improve the appearance of the eyes specifically and the face in a general way.

Upper eyelid fullness is a familial characteristic that is inherent from childhood. Surgery can produce surprising transformations and can be performed at any time after adolescence. On the other hand, excess skin of the upper eyelid is a laxity condition related to aging. Surgery produces a tightening effect especially favored by women because it allows them to wear eye make-up more effectively.

Lower eyelid fullness is also a familial characteristic, and may become more pronounced with age. Chronic allergies can worsen swelling of the eyelids. This condition can be improved substantially in both women and men, relieving the "tired" appearance.

Surgery is not truly effective in the improvement of lower eyelid wrinkles. The problem is that to remove all the wrinkles, generally too much skin has to be removed, causing the eyelid to pull downward. Another problem is that as the incisions heal, they may contract. If so, the eyelid margin may be pulled down and out causing a chronically dry and irritated eye from the excessive exposure. Chemical "peels" are more effective. When there are lower eyelid bags and wrinkles, the surgery for the bags is performed first, followed by chemical peeling for the wrinkles.

Blepharoplasty, also known as "eyelid lift," is the operation which improves the appearance of the eyes by removing excess skin and puffiness from the upper and lower eyelids. This procedure results in a more youthful and rested look, and can improve peripheral vision. There is an interesting sense of lessened fatigue and eye strain.

"Upper blepharoplasty" surgery on the upper eyelids is different for men than for women because of different objectives. In women, the removal of upper eyelid fullness aims to create a deepening of the normal upper eyelid crease and permit a more effective use of eye make-up to enhance the eyes. Surgery of the upper eyelid may produce very dramatic results (Fig. 14–7A and Fig. 14–7B).

The removal of excess skin also produces a "cleaner" appearance of the upper eyelid crease.

The goal of upper eyelid surgery in men is to produce a moderate reduction of excess skin, which sometimes overlaps the eyelashes and may even obstruct vision. Surgery must be moderate and subtle, to avoid an artificial or even feminine look.

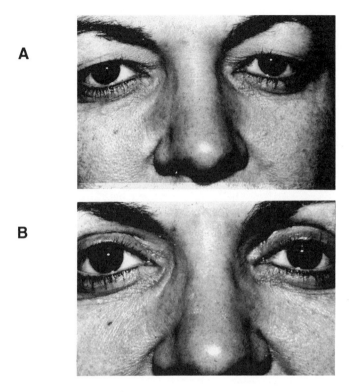

Figure 14–7 Upper blepharoplasty in female before and after surgical correction.
(A) Note the excess skin and bagginess of the upper eyelids.
(B) Cosmetic removal of excess skin in the upper eyelids of the woman enhances her upper eyelid appearance.

Lower blepharoplasty is the removal of bags from the lower eyelid and is one of the most successful cosmetic procedures in ophthalmic plastic surgery. It is commonly called "the surgery for executives" because so many of them request this surgery to achieve a younger, more vigorous appearance (Fig. 14–8A and Fig. 14–8B). The appearance of the eyes after recovery is so natural that people cannot tell that any surgery has been performed. Lower eyelid blepharoplasty is always considered a cosmetic surgery.

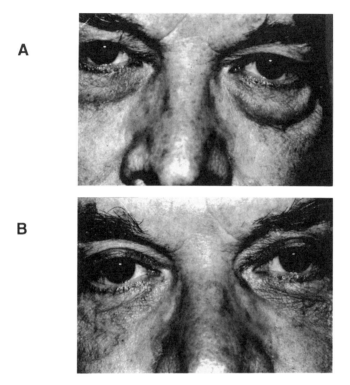

Figure 14–8 Before and after lower blepharoplasty, or "executive surgery" in men.
(A) Note the tired, worn-out look of this man caused by the excess lower eyelid bagginess and puffiness.
(B) "Executive surgery" in men is frequently used by prominent businessmen to effectively diminish a sluggish appearance.

Upper blepharoplasty is considered "medically necessary" when the overhanging skin obscures the vision or weighs on the eyelashes so that it turns the eyelashes down. When done solely for cosmetic purposes, the surgery is not insured and must be paid for by the patient.

Blepharoplasty takes approximately one hour and 30 minutes for all four eyelids, or approximately 50 minutes for upper eyelids or the lower eyelids. After a blepharoplasty, patients are allowed to go home, once fully awake. There are no bandages, so they are able, following surgery, to read or watch television. The day following surgery, some patients may be able to go back to work. Other patients prefer to remain in social isolation until the black and blue marks which may have resulted from surgery disappear. This occurs after approximately one week. Normal work activities, except for heavy exercise, may be resumed by the fourth day. On the eighth day, patients may resume heavy exercising such as jogging and aerobics. Pain is usually moderate and may be controlled by Tylenol™.

Conclusion

Whether to confront disease or to make the eyes more attractive, modern procedures are light years ahead of where they were a generation ago. Costs are down, effectiveness high, and time spent in discomfort inconsequential. What once was the domain of the rich can now be sought out by those with average incomes. Statistics tell us this is becoming the "norm."

Wrap-Up

- Normal eyelid positioning and tightness is necessary for healthy eyes and good vision.
- Ocuplastic surgery repairs cancerous diseased tissues, droopy or malpositioned tissues, or cosmetically unsightly tissues.
- Upper eyelid blepharoplasty is medically indicated when the upper eyelid droop interferes with vision, driving, and reading.
- Drooping of the eyelids is called ptosis. Ptosis may be an inherited natural aging change, a result of chronic eye rubbing, neurological or traumatic injury, or a result of excessively thick and heavy upper eyelid tissue.

- The repair of the lower eyelid is necessary if the eyelid begins to sag causing corneal exposure, or interference with tear drainage, or if the eyelid rolls outward or uncomfortably rolls inward.
- Skin cancers are very common on the face and eyelids. It is a localized invasive tumor.
- Squamous cell carcinomas are associated with excessive sun exposure and can be both locally invasive as well as spreading to regional lymph nodes.

Chapter Fifteen

Visible Drug Effects

Warren D. Cross

Many people are concerned today about substance abuse and its influence on social norms, ethics, and the economy. That the situation is as much a psychological and medical problem as a matter for law enforcement is beginning to be understood even in the most conservative quarters. Ophthalmologists are interested in the question, both as citizens hoping to make a difference, and as doctors who can offer information based upon their training.

Drugs of any sort influence the brain and its behavior, and this can be detected in that most valuable near accessory, the eye. Many drugs which alter brain activity by increasing or decreasing optical functioning will be visible and detectable in the eyes. Four of the 12 cranial nerves control vision, and eye and eyelid movement. Business organizations, no more effective than others who perform "policing" tasks, wonder about behavior patterns of employees or potential employees. Yes, personal inclinations are a private matter; but if they influence the success or failure of a corporation, or your job or safety as an employee, then you and the corporation have justification to learn about present or potential problems and to use that information in making personnel decisions.

Since the eye is a sensitive reflection of the brain's activity levels, it should be no surprise that an observant onlooker, knowing what eye signs to check, can spot dead giveaways revealing drug use. The

North American Institute (NAI) in Austin, Texas, has designed a five-step drug and alcohol test which is in part simplification of the basic office eye examination and in part the field sobriety test used by law enforcement officers for about four decades. Virtually any person can understand and perform it. OpticALERT™ can be used by law enforcement officers, personnel officers, employees, parents and teenagers, or anyone else who wants a quick, reliable means of spotting drug use without the trouble, expense, and legal problems of a body fluids analysis.

The five-step procedure is a basic application of everything you have learned in this book. The North American Institute has a complete program with excerpts as follows. While their "Five Step OpticALERT™" is invaluable and interesting, it is meant to be used in combination with "probable cause." Probable cause means, for example, that if your employee, child or spouse appears anxious or depressed and begins exhibiting lifestyle changes such as: making mental mistakes; changing friends; dressing sloppily; constantly wearing sunglasses; and generally becoming less effective in personal and business matters, you may suspect drugs and/or alcohol abuse.

In the NAI's experience, OpticALERT™ is correct 93 percent of the time in corporate and employee situations. You must have the individual's cooperation and the examination must be done in a quiet room. If the person is an employee, the legal steps to protect you and your company can be explained and must be documented. You should consult your attorney or the NAI. A careful explanation of OpticALERT™ to your children, along with the understanding that you will check them with this program if you are suspicious, will help make this a positive tool to reduce peer pressure. This awareness may help your child to "just say no" and save a life! Parents who discuss family values and express knowledge and concern about drug use can assist their children in their response to peer pressure. It becomes easier for your children to say, "I can't do that, my parents will know I did drugs." Statistics have shown that adolescents use drugs for two years before being discovered by their parents. NAI suggests leaving OpticALERT™ information on the corner of the kitchen cabinet, or where they will see it, to serve as a reminder.

Visible Drug Effects 251

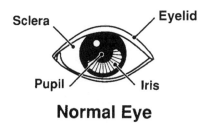

Normal Eye

Figure 15–1   A normal eye. The upper eyelid covers a small portion of the iris, but doesn't overlap the pupil. The pupil width itself is about the same size as one side of the iris. The sclera is white or buff and clear of redness.

To receive a positive finding, a person must fail two or more of the five steps in the test. Since the brain innervates and controls the eyes equally, the abnormal findings typically should be present and equal in both eyes.

Consider the normal eye (Fig. 15–1). The upper and lower eyelids cover a small part of the iris but do not normally droop or overlap the pupil. The iris, according to one's genetic inheritance, is a shade of either brown, blue, or green. The width of the pupil in normal light is usually about the same size as one side of the iris framed by the eyelids, or about one-third the total iris diameter. The sclera is white, or sometimes buff color, and should be clear of redness.

The first step of the OpticALERT™ examination is a quick general observation of the eye. Many commonly used drugs such as cocaine, marijuana, PCP, heroin, or even alcohol give the sclera a reddish coloration. A first thing to note is whether or not an individual's eye whites are actually reddish. Allergies, in season, can produce slight swelling and redness, and there will be water under the conjunctiva and other signs of seasonal allergy. Since they are balms, not substitutes for tears, continual use of either Visine™ or Murine™ eye drops, or Propine™ for glaucoma, may cause a similar redness of the eyes. Many drug users use these drops in an attempt to disguise their drug problem. If the eyes are red because of these eyedrops, the other steps should still be normal. Acute conjunctivitis or "pinkeye" does not last all year.

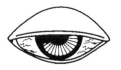

Droopy or Swollen Eyelid
Excessive Redness

Figure 15–2 A droopy or swollen eyelid with excessive redness. Cocaine, marijuana, alcohol, PCP, heroin, and other drugs cause the sclera to be red. When taken in high doses, these drugs make the eyelid swell, causing it to droop and touch the pupil.

"Droopy lids," sometimes sexistly referred to as "bedroom eyes" in young women, are usually present at birth. In some families the characteristic lingers on into adulthood. One certain way to maintain droop is to use drugs on a regular basis. This can make the ordinary eyelid swell or droop enough sometimes to touch the pupil (Fig. 15–2). Droopy eyelids that "happen" to rise and fall with coffee breaks and lunch hours may indicate drug use, and widely retracted eyelids especially can be caused by extensive cocaine abuse. Unless a person has severe thyroid disease, this unusual lid position can be a strong sign of drug use.

Next, the observer should look at the pupil. If it is either noticeably larger (Fig. 15–3A) or smaller (Fig. 15–3B) than should be the case in normal light, a history of drug use can be suspected. A ruler can be used in this part of the test. The pupil can range in size from 1.0 mm to 8.0 mm in diameter, but normal size is ordinarily less than that, about 3.0 mm to 6.0 mm. An enlarged pupil hints strongly at the presence of cocaine, marijuana, amphetamines, and the like. A tiny pupil suggests use of heroin, sedatives, and very high use of cocaine and marijuana. If only one pupil is dilated at the time of the test, there may be a neurological problem or a history of trauma. Pilocarpine™, a prescribed drug used to treat glaucoma, also produces pinpoint pupils, so the subject should be questioned about recent medical history when this condition is noticed. Both pupils

A

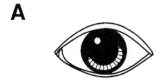

Dilated or Enlarged Pupil

B

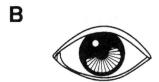

Tiny or Constricted Pupil

Figure 15–3 (A) A dilated or enlarged pupil in normal lighting is much larger than one side of the iris, and may suggest drug use such as cocaine, marijuana, and amphetamines.
(B) A constricted or tiny pupil in normal lighting is much smaller than one side of the iris, and suggests drug use such as heroin, sedatives, marijuana, and cocaine.

should move at the same rate. Some people naturally have a slight size differential between the pupils which is normal and is not a test failure.

The third step in this test requires use of a bright, directed light beam, the sort one finds in pen lights. The light is held about six inches away from the eye, aimed at the pupil, and brought in to within one inch. If normal, the pupil will contract rapidly; if hindered by drugs, the pupil will contract very slowly, or not at all (Fig. 15–4). This failure of the pupil to contract, incidentally, is one important reason why someone under the influence is a hazard if operating a vehicle or heavy equipment. In addition to judgment being impaired, without the pupil operating normally, one cannot as accurately estimate distance, depth, or dimensions.

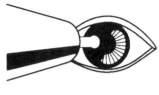

Light Check

Figure 15–4   The light check. In a normal eye, when a small penlight is held approximately six inches away and is shined into the eye, the eye rapidly constricts. Under the influence of drugs, the eye will shrink very slowly, if at all.

Next, the examiner watches horizontal eye tracking (Fig. 15–5). An object, perhaps the penlight used in step three of the test, is held upright about a foot in front of the eye. Keeping the head motionless, it is moved right and left to the most extreme point on which the eyes can train. Normal conditions permit tracking in a smooth motion and easily holding a gaze on the outmost point for several seconds. Abnormal conditions will show up as a jerky motion of the eyes while tracking, and difficulty in maintaining a focus at the margin of rotation.

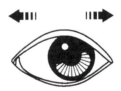

Eye Tracking

Figure 15–5   Eye tracking. In a sober individual, the normal eye can follow an object in a smooth motion with the head held still. Under the influence of drugs, the eye is unable to follow the object smoothly. The eye bounces or jerks while following the object, and has difficult holding a fixed gaze. Failure to track strongly indicates drug use.

Visible Drug Effects

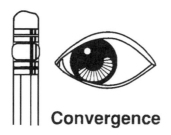

Convergence

Figure 15–6 Convergence. A person not under the influence of drugs can follow an object held six to eight inches from his eye and hold fixation of the object while it is brought toward his nose. Under severe drug influence, an individual can't even begin to cross his eyes and focus on the object. He may stare straight ahead fixedly.

This should not and could not be confused with a person who has *nystagmus* or "dancing eyes." This neurological problem causes eyes to move back and forth in any of several different motor patterns. Nystagmus should be in the medical history and could be confirmed by an eye doctor.

The final part of the examination for drugs is another kind of tracking test (Fig. 15–6). The individual's head is tilted to about 45 degrees and a focal object is presented at about six inches away. It is brought in close, and the effort to focus is observed. Unless drugs are being used, a person can track the diminishing focal length easily; otherwise, the task is difficult and the eyes will tend to drift back to a greater focal point. If an individual is really "hammered," he won't even be able to start a cross-eyed focus. The tester should make certain that the subject does not have a history of convergence deficiency, which produces the same effect without drug use.

A strong positive indication from both eyes of failing two or more steps in the OpticALERT™ test should be verified through a standard body fluids test. The eye check cannot distinguish between legal and illegal drugs. You should be aware if a person is taking prescription medication or over-the-counter medication.

Abnormal eyes may simply reflect genetic inheritance or a medical condition, but for most people they are a dead give-away.

For further information, please call or write:

North American Institute
5918 Courtyard Drive, Fifth Floor
Austin, TX 78730
(512) 338-4644

In the case of emergencies, contact:

Alcohol and Drug Referral Hot Line: 1-800-252-6465
Child's Help—National Child Abuse Hot Line: 1-800-422-4453
National Cocaine Hot Line: 1-800-262-2463

Wrap-Up

- The eyes are a sensitive reflection of the brain's activity.
- Four of the 12 cranial nerves control our vision, focusing, and eye movements.
- Drugs of any sort, legal or illegal, influence the brain and its behavior.
- Alcohol is two times greater a problem in the workplace than drugs.
- OpticALERT™ uses a five-step procedure to evaluate the level of brain activity.
- When the five steps are used in conjunction with probable cause, for example, changes in dress or friends, or increased mental mistakes, the five-step program is accurate over 90 percent of the time.
- The five steps of the OpticALERT™ program are:
    1. General observation of the eyes.
    2. Observation of the pupil size.
    3. Pupillary reaction to light.
    4. Horizontal eye tracking.
    5. Convergence ability.

- Tests of bodily fluids, such as blood and urine, is the only 100 percent positive test.
- Legal rights must be observed and protected at work and may be instrumental in family situations.

Chapter Sixteen

Ocular Emergencies

Warren D. Cross

Man's upright, two-legged stance permitted the development of a critically important relationship between the hands, the eyes, and the brain function. Remove any part of this unique set of components and you have a completely different creature. Losing our sight is highly traumatic. Cut us off from the visual world and you destroy a great part of our survival capacity and ability to enjoy life.

Partial or total loss of vision is always a possibility in life and considered an ocular emergency. Any number of things can happen to our eyes. Some traumas can be associated with great discomfort while others are undramatic and gradual. However they evolve, becoming familiar with the major causes of eyesight impairment and the symptoms that accompany them is a first step to the recognition of a problem and successful treatment thereof. Nearly everyone has heard of *retinal detachment.* Most patients assume that if they cannot see, they must have a retinal detachment. At the moment, the incidence of retinal detachment in the developed world varies between eight and 18 cases per 100,000 per year. The initial signs of retinal detachment are varied. The individual may notice flashes of light when the eye moves quickly, or become aware of black "floaters," similar to pepper, in the field of vision. Most of us have or will experience the gray irregularly shaped floaters associated with aging changes in the vitreous. Black floaters are red blood cells or clumps of red blood cells associated with a retinal tear or hemorrhage inside your eye. Other symptoms of a retinal detachment may be that of the appearance of a "lacy veil" or "curtain" coming across your vision from the outside, or the loss of a portion of your peripheral vision. Should you feel you have a retinal detachment, a way to determine in which eye the retinal detachment is located is to cover the eyes alternately. Whatever the symptoms, the condition is painless. Those especially at risk for retinal detachment frequently have family histories of this problem. The odds of this condition developing increase with nearsightedness and age, and with any significant blows to the face. If detachment occurs in one eye, there is about a 25 percent chance of detachment occurring in the other eye.

An eye can become blind due to any of several blood problems. A painless blockage in an eye's arteries or veins may be immediately noticeable, for vision could drop to the point of only perceiving imageless light. Diseases involving the blood such as *diabetes mellitus* and *atheromatous vascular plaques* can produce localized blockages in the arteries and veins of the retina also. Inflammation of the blood vessels called *vasculitis* associated with the autoimmune diseases such as arthritis and lupus are frequent causes of sudden blindness. This is frequently associated with inflamed vessels in the temple area called *temporal-arteritis*. Blood diseases, high blood pressure, and aging can produce damage to the macula and cause either gradual or sudden loss of vision at the center of the visual field.

Vitreous hemorrhage, or bleeding into the vitreous body, is a painless yet serious condition. Vitreous hemorrhages have many causes, including diabetes, retinal tears, hypertension, surgery, trauma, and tumors. If you suffer a vitreous hemorrhage, do not lift any heavy objects until you see your ophthalmologist. If the blood is in the anterior chamber it is referred to as a *hyphema*. The blood may be the result of surgery, or blunt trauma. The blood in either chamber will slowly be absorbed and clear the vision, unless the source of the bleeding continues to leak. Since blood is thicker than the aqueous fluid, *traumatic glaucoma* is possible.

For athletes and other individuals who participate in energetic activity, the *blunt trauma* of blows to the eye is a frequent cause of

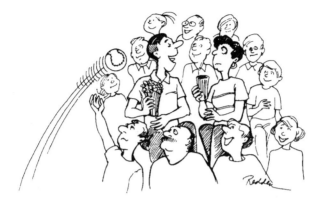

Figure 16–1 Loquacious man in stands turns to talk to wife. Batter on baseball field far below has just hit a foul ball which is streaking toward the unattentive man's face.

blindness (Fig. 16–1). The eye is recessed into its orbit and protected by bone and tissue, but direct impacts or shocks from the head being hit from any angle can produce damage. "Shiners," a result of bleeding into the fat and muscle around the eye, which look terrible and require cold packs, can hint at deeper problems such as a cracked orbital wall. If this is the case, the injured eye may be unable to track in parallel with the uninjured eye, and surgery may be necessary to correct matters. This problem is commonly referred to as a *blow out fracture*. Blows can also produce scratches on the front of the eye, a tearing of the iris, a bursting of one or the other of the eye chambers, a ripping of the optic nerve, or retinal tears. The natural lens can also be torn loose or can develop into a cataract condition.

Cuts or punctures of the eye can result from any sharp object, ranging from pencils, to fish hooks, to animal teeth. In severe injuries, the eyelids may be lacerated as well as the cornea and the eyeball. In this situation, extreme care must be exercised to avoid applying pressure or manipulating the tissues of the wounded eye. A light sterile dressing and/or possibly a rigid shield is the best precaution. Do not attempt to remove the offending fish hook, pen, stick, or invasive object.

If the foreign object is not embedded in the eye, bring the object with you for the ophthalmologist to examine at his office or at the hospital Emergency Room. Do not eat or drink after the injury. If surgical repair is required, surgery may be delayed if you have recently eaten. These injuries are as terrible as they sound, yet generation after generation of young men continue to risk their sight in ill-conceived altercations in road houses or as professional boxers in the ring. If they knew what they were risking, they might not put up their "dukes" so fast.

Modern life offers plenty of chemical hazards that harm the eye. The possibilities are endless, and can occur without warning. A car battery explodes, the pepper sauce for blackened redfish flashes into white smoke filling the kitchen, a sneeze puffs an alkaline cleanser into your face, a dropped bottle of ammonia splashes up on you . . . The possibilities are endless.

Intelligent prevention dictates the use of safety glasses whenever there is the slightest chance of an acid, solvent, or other chemical becoming a danger. Caustic chemicals must be locked and secured from children, and children should be cautioned as to what might happen to cause a serious accident. If chemicals should get into the eyes, they should be flushed immediately with water for at least 15 minutes (Fig. 16–2). Following this, an immediate trip to a doctor for treatment is always warranted. If possible, bring information regarding the chemical which got into the eye since treatment varies from chemical to chemical.

More tangible material can get into the eyes. In our dirty cities the air is filled with soot, dust and pollen. Rocks and gravel spray from road shoulders, sand falls from concrete trucks, nails are flipped up and at you. Motorized lawn equipment flings dirt and chopped grass, grinders and saws hurl metal and wood shavings. The minor particles can be washed out with tears or water, or contact lens saline solutions. If a particle remains in the eye, it should not be removed with a Q-tip under any circumstances. See your doctor immediately.

The eyes are affected by many diseases, such as acute angle closure glaucoma as discussed in Chapter Seven. Another example may be *optic neuritis,* an inflammatory or autoimmune problem in

Ocular Emergencies

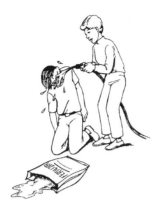

Figure 16–2 Man kneels on lawn as his wife pours water on his open injured eye.

which there is reduced nerve conduction, decreased vision, and discomfort in movement of the eye which can be caused by multiple sclerosis. If the sinuses become infected or you develop a severe stye, *orbital cellulitis,* a progressive redness and swelling of the soft tissues around the eye, can be prevalent. The person will find dimming vision, eye swelling, reddening of the conjunctiva, and severe pain when the eye is rotated. The infection is quite serious, and may even spread to the brain.

Ophthalmic poisons can cause a loss of vision resulting from industrial chemicals such as methyl alcohol (wood alcohol) and halogens. Certain drugs, especially the phenothiazines and plaquenil, may also cause decreased vision.

Ultraviolet light is the most common offender that causes radiant energy injuries and decreased vision. Such conditions as "welder's burn," "snow burn," and the popular "tanning salon burn" are the most frequent sources of radiant eye injuries. Ultraviolet light causes ultraviolet keratitis by killing the epithelial cells on the surface of the cornea causing pain, tearing, light sensitivity, and poor vision. These symptoms generally last about 24 hours. Until professional help can be obtained, artificial tears such as CelluviscTM and significant oral doses of ibuprofen should alleviate the discomfort.

If you focus directly on ultraviolet sources of light or the sun without the proper protective eye wear, you may permanently burn or injure the macula with serious visual changes.

Any consistent and persistent change in a pupil or eyelid position should be reported to your eye doctor. If accompanied by a headache, an Emergency Room situation could exist which would require a careful diagnosis.

The sudden onset of "two different images at the same time" which lasts for more than several seconds, should be checked. These symptoms are often associated with recent blunt head trauma or a fall causing edema or injury of a nerve controlling the eye or a sudden bleed similar to one that President Reagan experienced. Most commonly, it is associated with diabetes and/or hypertension. Cerebral vascular accidents and tumors should also be considered.

If a cerebral stroke affects the area of the brain which controls your vision, there exists a possibility that all or part of your vision may be absent. Occasionally, the stroke is localized, affecting only your vision so that you may have very few other symptoms such as inability to talk or move an extremity.

Metamorphopsia describes the distortion or "stretching," and compression or minification (making smaller) of the macula that develops when fluid from a cyst or a hemorrhage increases the intraocular eye pressure. This condition becomes more common with increasing age and a known history of macular degeneration. Ophthalmic care should be sought as soon as possible.

Corneal ulcers and corneal herpetic keratitis are always serious. For example, if you are a contact lens wearer and you develop pain, discharge, light sensitivity and a red eye with decreasing vision, you must see your doctor immediately (Chapter Eleven).

No discussion about sudden loss or change of vision could be complete without mentioning *hysterical blindness*. Hysterical blindness can be difficult to diagnose as well as to prove. Clever neurological "tricks" are needed to diagnose this condition. A person suspected of hysteria may need psychiatric treatment to help in the understanding of his problem.

Two of the less frequent illnesses of the eye are *rubeosis* of the iris and the various forms of *uveitis*.

Rubeosis is the proliferation of small, fine vessels in the inside of the eye and is associated with numerous conditions such as diabetes mellitus or may follow closure of the central retinal vein. New blood vessels spontaneously appear on the surface of the iris, especially near the pupil. If unchecked, vision may become reduced due to retinal changes. Hemorrhages of blood vessels into the frontal chamber can also occur. This may lead to types of glaucoma which are difficult to fight by medical or surgical means. Rubeosis seems to follow episodes of radiation therapy exposure, artery and vein blockages, intraocular inflammations of the uveitis type, and other abnormalities.

Uveitis is a term covering a widespread group of inflammatory disorders of the uveal region of the eye—the iris, ciliary body, choroid, retina, optic nerve, and vitreous body—all of which are nourished by blood from a common artery. Depending upon which tissue is inflamed or infected, the condition is named by adding the suffix "itis" to the name of the tissue. So we have "iritis," "cyclitis," "iridocyclitis" (inflammation of the iris and ciliary body), "choroiditis," "chorioretinitis" (inflammation of the choroid and retina), or "panuveitis" or "enophthalmitis" (inflammation of all the parts).

The inflammation may be sterile, or possess no bacteria. Uveitis is similar to the inflammations we get in our joints which is called "arthritis"—similar to an arthritis of the eye. All such inflammations have a high association with the autoimmune diseases, especially rheumatoid arthritis, lupus, and Crohn's disease. Other inflammations result from fungi, viruses such as herpes simplex, rubella, or the cytomegalic inclusion disease often associated with Acquired Immune Deficiency Syndrome (AIDS). Some sources of uveitis are within the eye itself, such as a "leaking" cataract, necrosis of an intraocular tumor, or reactions to other problems.

Non-sterile inflammations of the eye are most commonly produced by bacteria growing in the eye. The bacteria may enter the eye as a result of injury, such as a corneal laceration or perforation, a corneal ulcer, and even surgical incisions following surgical procedures. Rarely does the eye become infected by transmission of bacteria from inside the body such as from a diseased lung or kidney.

Signs and symptoms of uveitis include increased light sensitivity, progressive redness of the eye, and progressive decreases in vision. Such symptoms demand immediate examination and treatment. The first thing is to discover what type of inflammation is involved. Then every effort must be made to apply a high concentration of the right medications needed to kill the organism. Since there are so many possible culprits and so much analysis needed to make a precise identification, time frequently does not allow more than an estimate as to a diagnosis. Usually, diseases are initially treated by broad-spectrum antibiotics given either topically, subconjunctivally (injected into the thin outer covering of the eye), or systemically (injected into the body or taken in pill or capsule form). Drugs such as corticosteroids and non-steroidal anti-inflammatory medications are frequently prescribed if uveitis is sterile.

If the inflammation destroys the eye in spite of all the combative efforts, much or all of the eye may need to be removed. If the scleral shell is left, the operation is called *evisceration*"; if the entire eye is removed, the operation is called *enucleation.* Usually neither is a genuine prospect, so long as the problem is addressed quickly.

The bottom line on emergencies is to remain aware of your eyes, noting any changes in your vision or how your eye looks or feels. Bleedings or leaks in the eye fluid are obvious signs of a need for treatment, as is reddening, discharge, pain, light sensitivity, blank spots in the field of vision and the swelling of the eye itself. With a delicate organ such as the eye, it is better to get an examination as early as possible if anything seems amiss, for a slight problem can rapidly turn into a major problem.

Wrap-Up

- When in a situation that could be injurious to your eyes, such as using lawn care equipment and power tools, or playing racquetball, or exposure to radiant energy (UV, infrared, X-ray, lasers), always wear wraparound goggles specially designed to protect you from these dangers.

- Any sudden or progressive loss of vision in either one or both eyes should be a reason to see your ophthalmologist as soon as possible.
- Any chemicals splashed into the eyes should immediately be irrigated or flushed with water or other appropriate solutions for 15 minutes minimum. Then see your ophthalmologist. Bring the solution label or bottle with you if possible.
- Follow your doctor's instructions regarding use of all eye medications, and check expiration dates. Be sure all medications and solutions used are labeled "ophthalmic." This indicates the drugs are of a correct pH and concentration for use in the eyes.
- If irrigation is not successful to remove a foreign body, *do not* attempt to remove the foreign body yourself.
- Flashes of light, visual distortions, headaches, light sensitivity, discharge, double vision, redness or pain in the eye are all indications to see your ophthalmologist immediately.

Chapter Seventeen

Understanding Insurance

Joseph Fitzgerald and Pamela Pullings

Today there are many controversial issues surrounding health care, not the least of which involves how to pay and how much to pay for services rendered. Since each health care plan and insurance policy is different, persons trying to make an informed decision about which plan is best for them can find studying alternatives frustrating, to say the least. This chapter will provide a better understanding of how current insurance plans work. Much of the greater part of medical work done on the eyes can be covered by one source of insurance or another, but only if insurance is used.

When the notion of insurance first got started at Lloyd's of London, a seventeenth-century ale house and gaming den, it started as wagers about whether or not, or when, ships plying international waters would arrive safely at the Port of London. Gradually this informal system of bets, second-guesses, and estimates of navigational hazards developed into a situation in which statistics of occurrence were tabulated by certain sharp-eyed gentlemen with a penchant for numbers. Those who were best at the game eventually went into the business on a full-time basis. They called themselves "carriers" in fond remembrance of the old days when they "carried bets." The term has stuck, and all insurance corporations, whether involved in life, property, or any other kind of insurance, refer to themselves as *carriers* to the present day.

Terms used in this chapter are clarified below so you may have a better understanding of the insurance definitions referred to in the following pages. Some of these terms may have two applicable definitions when referring to insurance.

An *allowance* is the fee amount for a service which is regarded as reasonable and customary. One would expect that in a rational world this amount would be the same everywhere, but such is not the case. Since the world we have to live in is arbitrary and capricious, the value has a lot to do with overhead produced by local economic conditions. Allowance amounts vary from insurance carrier to insurance carrier and from locality to locality.

Assignment has two meanings. In one sense, assignment refers to the decision about whether or not payment of benefits will be sent directly to the service provider, such as the doctor or hospital, or sent directly to the person who received the service—you. If you want benefits to be sent directly to the provider by your insurance company, written authorization is needed. All insurance claim forms have a place for this routing of funds to be authorized by signature.

The other meaning of assignment relates value to the insurance carrier's position on how much it will actually pay for a service. Payment might be in full if its auditors agree with local notions of a fair allowance. Commonly, the astute wielders of fiduciary ethics employed by the insurance carrier regard allowances as way too high, or call one's attention to fine print in the policy which limit payments to a percentage of assigned value, however reached. Frequently, the outcome is that they pay only a part of what is owed, leaving a balance for which the individual or another insurance company may be liable.

Every money payment is called a *benefit*. Each benefit is paid according to your policy's provisions, terms, and limitations. Routine eye exams are generally not a benefit. Frequently, your examination must be associated with a problem, such as pain, a cataract, glaucoma, or a foreign body in the eye.

Which brings us to *co-insurance*. The *primary carrier* is the first insurance company responsible for payment against services rendered. Consumer encounters with unresponsive insurance carriers over the past couple of centuries have revealed a consistent tendency to recalculate servicers' value estimations at a moderate or considerably lower level. That gap, and the inevitable deductible clauses, has meant that many people add another carrier or two for only a segment of coverage, to be on the safe side. These *secondary carriers* can be contracted at any scale of coverage. Claims are sent to them after an explanation of benefits is received from the primary carrier. By law, all carriers have to define what services they will or will not pay for. These are called *covered expenses,* more jargon derived from the days when "bets were covered."

The *deductible* is an idiosyncratic out-of-pocket expense for the insured person, an amount specified by each carrier according to its own perspectives. Once you have paid the deductible amount for any calendar year, additional loss is covered by the carrier. The deductible is not due again until the next calendar year begins, unless otherwise specified by your insurance policy.

The *effective date of policy* is the basepoint after which the carrier has an obligation to adhere to the terms of coverage. After that point, during the defined period of the policy, the carrier must give reimbursement, albeit as anemic as possible.

An important way insurance carriers stay solvent is to include policy provisions which define certain sorts of services so that the carriers won't have to pay on them if the policy holder gets the service done. These *exclusions* can be pretty tricky, and take some careful reading to ferret out. If a policy holder finds something "iffy" after signing, forget about getting anything changed until the policy is renewed. After all, a bet is a bet.

While many services are excluded outright, *policy provisions* specify exactly what will not be covered unless exact, defined conditions exist. This is also highly important to keep the carrier's profit and loss relationship under control. Eye exams, eyeglasses, and pregnancy are often a policy provision.

When a carrier finally pays for services, its invoice includes an *explanation of benefits,* or "E.O.B." This is a detailed, itemized listing of the charges that were submitted, the dollar amounts considered for payment, applicable deductions, and the amount of actual payments that will be made.

If you have a *pre-existing condition,* something for which medical help was given prior to signing a contract with an insurance carrier, the policy petitioner is an obvious bad risk. Usually, if a treatment or diagnosis was made within three months of the effective date of a new policy, the carrier will not cover this condition for a period of six months to two years, depending on the policy. The naive beware: If the insurance carrier has defined itself like this, the patient will be responsible for the entire amount charged for a service relating to a pre-existing condition.

A *participating provider* is a medical doctor or entity who has signed an agreement or contract with an insurance carrier. This frequently has to do either with an agreed-upon allowance or with some sort of flat rate group coverage the carrier has negotiated.

The amount a carrier considers to be the maximum allowance for a submitted charge is always called *reasonable and customary,* harking for legitimacy back to Anglo-Saxon tenets of common law. If the carrier quibbles that the total amount charged by your provider is over the amount it claims is reasonable and customary in your locality, the provider may bill you for the difference. This nasty shock is getting to be less frequent, since many providers have signed contracts with the insurance carriers in which they agree to accept the carriers' reasonable and customary charges as the maximum amount for which they will bill or attempt to collect.

Now that we have the basic terms straight, we can move ahead and discuss the broad picture of health insurance and how it can be used to take care of your eyes' medical needs.

Health insurance is primarily obtained through employers' policies, with conditions worked out between management and either unions or union-like organizations of workers. This kind of coverage is called *group health insurance.* Some larger companies may present a menu of several alternative insurance plans to choose from. Insider insurance agent jargon refers to these as "cafeteria" plans. Whichever plan you choose, the employer generally pays a portion of the monthly premium due on your behalf and deducts the balance from the worker's payroll check as needed. Usually, additional coverage for spouses and children is available at an additional cost.

Anyone not fortunate enough to have group health insurance as an option can either seek public assistance, or line up an individual policy through the insurance carrier of their choice. The selection had best be carefully made, with considerable attention paid to all explicitly spelled out provisions. A policy may hold a provision that excludes a service one needs or wishes to have.

Usually the potential outlay for coverage will be higher than in a group plan, since no economies of scale are involved for the carrier. One good way to hold down costs is to select a higher deductible and/or a higher co-insurance rate and not worry about the small expenses which may come up. Insurance should be considered coverage for calamities, not broken windows. Questions also need to be asked regarding pre-existing conditions, such as what time limitations there are on pre-existing conditions of coverage.

A retired military service person is probably covered under Champus insurance. If care is to be obtained outside a base medical facility, the former service person should make certain to contact Champus and learn if the policy covers payment to off-base physicians and/or facilities *before* the services are rendered.

For those who are not employed, or cannot afford to pay premiums on an individual policy, coverage may be obtained through a state-funded program, such as Medicaid in the State of Texas and MediCal in the State of California. Each state has a different name for this type of coverage which allows services for medical, dental, and vision care to qualified applicants. The Department of Health and Human Services/Resources in each state is the agency to contact for an appointment or application.

The federal government's Supplemental Security Income (SSI) is offered to people who don't qualify for the state-funded program but need financial and/or medical assistance. Either Health and Human Services or the local Social Security office is where to seek out information about this type of plan.

Once someone reaches the age of eligibility for federal medical benefits, Medicare becomes every American's primary carrier unless an income is being derived, not from a retirement plan, but from outright work, even part-time. In that case, the employer's group health plan remains the primary insurer. Those who continue to work after Medicare benefits become available must notify both Medicare and any private health insurance carriers of the situation so that benefits will be paid properly for all health care. Applying for and receiving your eligibility for Medicare benefits through the local Social Security office does not guarantee that claims will be paid properly or with dispatch. Also, it takes longer for Medicare benefits to be reimbursed the first time a Medicare claim is filed on your behalf. This is because the claim goes through a verification process before benefits are actually paid.

When a provider of services signs an agreement with Medicare stating he will provide services to Medicare eligible patients, he is obligated to follow Medicare's rules and guidelines. If the provider of service has not signed such an agreement with Medicare, the decision to accept a Medicare assignment is optional and moves into the realm of a mutual agreement between provider and the patient.

Medicare has its own annual deductible that must be paid at the beginning of each calendar year before benefits will be paid by Medicare for services rendered. After the individual meets the deductible, Medicare is obligated to pay 80 percent of all approved sums owed for treatments. For example, on a participating provider claim, where the total bill is $1,000.00 and Medicare's approved amount is $800.00, Medicare will make a payment of $640.00 (80 percent of the approved amount) to the provider of service. The patient is responsible for paying the difference of the amount which was approved, but not paid by Medicare—$160.00. Medicare has notified participating physicians that they are to collect this percentage and not the balance for the actual full amount billed.

Medicare will pay for an eye exam by an ophthalmologist or optometrist for the diagnosis or treatment of an infection, disease, or eye problem. Medicare does not pay for routine eye examinations. Medicare will allow payment for one lens in a pair of glasses for each eye that has undergone cataract surgery. This allowance is one lens per eye per lifetime.

Supplemental insurance payment can be solicited from the insurance carrier along with an explanation of Medicare benefits.

Many supplemental insurance carriers have agreed to participate in what is called "Medigap." This automatically forwards the Medicare claim to the supplemental insurance carrier for processing and payment and the paper work for elderly patients and their doctors.

Any office, clinic, or supplier of Medicare-approved services is required to file Medicare claims for their patients, regardless of whether they have signed the agreement of payment participation with Medicare. It is up to the individual provider of service as to whether the supplemental or secondary insurance policy will be filed by the physician's office or by the patient himself. Any physician's insurance officer can clarify where they stand on this issue.

If the supplemental insurance does not pay the 20 percent amount which is due, the patient is responsible for payment. Most supplemental insurance plans carry a separate deductible, which is not included in the annual Medicare deductible. This means the policy holder has to pay the deductible amount before benefits will be paid to the provider of service. Many dollars are wasted each year by senior citizens who invest innocently but futilely in "secondary insurance" that does not pay the percent that Medicare approves and is not really supplemental insurance. A secondary insurance policy is just another policy of the same kind. All Medicare patients obtaining additional insurance should be certain that the insurance is a *supplemental* policy to the Medicare and *not* a *secondary* policy.

Other obnoxious possible attributes of secondary or supplemental insurance plans are high deductible rates that must be paid in addition to the Medicare deductible. Also misleading can be the question of whether or not this supplemental insurance picks up the entire 20 percent of Medicare's approved amount. Some policies cover and pay only 80 percent of the *covered* 20 percent allowable! Again, a hard look at the fine print is always a good idea.

Many people are given a retirement package by their company which includes some sort of continuation of health care coverage. These are usually just secondary insurance packages that pay only if Medicare does not. The patient thinks that he has a supplemental policy and doesn't realize the difference until he receives an unexpected bill. Retirees need to ask their companies to redefine retirement insurance coverage as *supplemental, not secondary!*

When the elderly simply cannot afford to pay for additional insurance to cover the dreaded 20 percent, Medicare does allow providers of service to waive it on an individual basis. The provider of service, not the patient, must determine what is known as a *state of indigency*, grounds asserting that the patient does not have any other source of payment (e.g., Title XIX, a local welfare agency, a guardian, or other insurance) which would enable them to pay the amount initially billed. The provider of service must document that the cost of billing for and/or collecting the coinsurance/deductibles for a particular service exceeds or is disproportionate to the amounts to be collected. It's all more red tape for and from Uncle Sam.

Another avenue of health care coverage is through a *Health Maintenance Organization* (HMO). This organization provides a wide range of comprehensive health care services for a specified group at a fixed pre-arranged price. The choices are limited as to what kind of health care provider and type of service the patient can choose from. Enrollment in an HMO plan means assignment to a Primary Care Physician (PCP). This physician is chosen from an approved list. The purpose behind a PCP being assigned is so that overall care of a patient can be monitored, a function sometimes referred to as that of a "gate keeper." The PCP sees the individual first, then if necessary refers him to an in-area specialist.

Similar to the HMO plans are the *Preferred Provider Organization* (PPO) plans. A PPO contracts a group of primary care and specialist physicians. Most of the time patients have no PCP; instead, patients draw from a list of participating physicians in the PPO network for their health care needs. Some plans may have an individual and annual deductible which must be paid at the beginning of each year. Once the deductible has been satisfied, payment is probably only a percentage of services rendered, or a co-payment amount for each visit. Just because a doctor's name is listed in the PPO directory does not mean that a given insurance plan covers all services to that physician, such as routine eye exams from an eye doctor.

Everyone who gets into such an organization should make sure that they know whether or not a referral or pre-authorization is required for treatment, and if the service is covered under the policy. This should be learned before an office visit, diagnostic test, or surgical procedure is rendered. Many times, unfortunately, the PCP has not fully educated himself on the rules and regulations of each policy, and may not follow the channel of requirements to enable services to be reimbursed to the provider of service. Even in an emergency situation, the pre-certification is usually a requirement.

Many areas have developed another form of health care known as either *Independent Provider Associations* (IPA) or *Independent Provider Organizations* (IPO). These consist of groups of physicians and hospitals that provide a service similar to that of an HMO. Those individuals who join are assigned to a PCP, who in turn refers them to specialists, as needed. The IPA/IPOs contract with insurance companies. Physicians are not reimbursed on a fee-for-service basis, and payment is determined from a percentage of the total number of patients enrolled in the plan. The physicians are pre-paid for services, whether or not they see any or all of the enrolled members, an amount ranging from $0.75 to $15.00 per patient per month.

This has been compared to a form of "socialized medicine." The only difference is that the insurance companies in America are private, whereas in Canada the process is governmental.

Insurance carriers in the past have collected on premiums from their policy holders in advance, but paid out only after being billed for the services. In this situation the patient is given a plan where he is responsible only for the co-payment for each visit to the doctor's office or hospital, a payment ranging from $3.00 to $20.00. The physician gets paid a set amount, even if a catastrophe keeps him working 16 hours a day for weeks. For this reason, this type of plan is a good deal more popular with patients than with physicians.

Wrap-Up

- Insurance policies can and will be deceiving. Read and decipher the fine print before signing on the dotted line.

- Discuss your financial obligations with the eye doctor's insurance department before making your appointment so that you will know what you are up against financially.
- Know that the "best price" for a service does not always guarantee the "best results." New and inexperienced physicians may sometimes lower the cost for a surgery to get more patients to come in. Do not let yourself be a statistical review of their experience!
- Call the Better Business Bureau or State Board of Insurance to check out the reputation of your potential or existing insurance company.
- Always check your doctor's bill against the EOB, Explanation of Benefits, from your insurance company for accuracy. Everyone makes mistakes now and again.
- Estimates of common ophthalmological procedures:

  Reflects Surgeon Fee:

Cataract surgery	$1,500–2,600
Glaucoma surgery	$1,200–2,000
Corneal transplant	$2,300–2,800
Radial keratotomy	$ 600–1,200
Eyelid surgery for treatment of ptosis	$1,400–2,800

  Prices shown are an approximate cost per eye.

- Ophthalmological or optometric office visits/tests.

Annual eye exam	$ 60– 90
Six-month follow-up	$ 40– 65
Visual field testing	$ 40–100
A-scan calculations	$ 90–180
Fluorescein angiogram	$110–200
Contact lens fitting	$ 30– 70
Contact lens purchase	$ 25–200

Chapter Eighteen

Frequently Asked Questions

Warren D. Cross and Lawrence Lynn

Many patients visit an ophthalmologist (or any other medical specialist) and become frustrated. An important question was not answered, or the patient was reluctant to ask questions at all. It is helpful to both you and your doctor to make a list of questions and concerns before your visit. This list will enable your doctor to treat your condition more efficiently and help alleviate any anxiety you may be experiencing.

Two major ophthalmic clinics in Houston collected and collated questions asked by patients. The most frequently asked questions and answers were obtained from this questionnaire. We then reviewed the possible questions and selected the most appropriate responses. Some of the questions may be appropriate to your own situation or that of a friend, spouse, or child.

Ophthalmic Examinations

1. *How long does a comprehensive eye examination take?*
   The examination lasts one to two hours.

2. *How long will my eyes be dilated?*
   Your eyes will be dilated from about 30 minutes to four hours, depending upon the type of dilating drop used and your sensitivity to the drop.

3. *Can you speed up the "un-dilating" process by some suitable medication?*
   Yes, but it is best to let nature take its course. If you are uncomfortable under dilation, tell your doctor about it prior to dilation. He may use a milder dilating drop. Dapiprazole hydrochloride (Rev Eyes™) is occasionally used to reverse the dilation.

4. *Can I drive home, or back to my job, after the examination?*
   If you wait for the dilation to begin to diminish, yes. It is better to have another person drive you home or to work after a dilated examination. Driving with dilated eyes may be more difficult due to greater light sensitivity while the iris is open. Also, in younger individuals, dilation causes difficulty in close-up vision. Whether you drive or not, dark glasses should be worn (and are usually provided to you at the doctor's office) to decrease your light sensitivity.

5. *I use eyedrops to "take the red out," but I have heard that they are bad for my eyes. Is this true?*
   Over-the-counter drops are designed only for occasional use, no more than four or five times a month. If you use them every day your eyes will become habituated to them. Your eyes will then become red and irritated when the eyedrops are *not* present. Another reason to avoid these drops is because the chemicals in the over-the-counter eyedrops produce an antihistamine effect, and dry your eyes even further.

   Your doctor will prescribe steroid eyedrops and gradually reduce the dosage if the abuse of "whitening" eyedrops requires treatment. If you have significant allergies, newer products such as Ocular™, Alomide™, or Livostin™ may be prescribed by your doctor. The itching and swelling of the eyes may be relieved by ice compresses. A careful examination of your environment may be useful since some soaps and cleansers, hand lotions, make-up, cat and dog hair and dander, and other sources of irritation may be affecting your eye comfort. Frequent changes of household air filters, even upgrading your air filter to electrostatic filters, or to 3M Filtrete™, may help. Cheap fiberglass filters generally only filter out the worst allergy-stimulating dust and pollen.

Cataract Surgery

1. *Can't the cataract just be scraped off?*
   No. The cataract must be surgically removed.

2. *How soon can I go back to work after cataract surgery?*
   Often you can return to light work the next day after a cataract surgery and placement of an intraocular lens implant.

3. *How soon after cataract surgery can I lift heavy things, or get involved in strenuous activities, such as sex?*
   You should wait at least three weeks before engaging in strenuous activity or the lifting of heavy objects. Unstrenuous sex can be resumed in three days.

4. *Can't the cataract be eliminated with a laser?*
   Not at this time. Primary cataract extraction is like the extraction of a tooth. Lasers are used for minor follow-up surgeries.

5. *Does cataract surgery hurt?*
   You will only feel a mild sting from the very fine needle which provides the anesthetic. This is administered after you have been sedated. Most patients are amazed at the painlessness of cataract surgery. Some surgeons today are performing painless surgery on selected patients with only topical anesthetic eyedrops, amazing as it sounds.

6. *Will my vision be clear or blurry after cataract surgery?*
   Assuming the surgery has been properly performed, which happens in approximately 99 percent of all cases, you may have blurred vision for anywhere from one day to two weeks following surgery. Thereafter, your vision will be clear. You will be

amazed at the many things you can now see, how vivid and bright colors and objects really are!

7. *How soon can I get my new eyeglasses (if I need any) after cataract surgery?*
   It's best to wait at least one to two months if possible before buying new prescription lenses. Your eye and its vision need time to stabilize.

Refractive Surgery

1. *Cutting the surface of the eye suggests a lot of pain. How badly does this surgery hurt?*
   The surgery itself is painless. You should feel no pain before or during surgery because topical anesthetics are used, and the level of anesthesia is carefully maintained during surgery. Until about two years ago, the effects of the anesthetic would last for at least an hour or two after surgery, then patients would feel a significant amount of pain unless they were diligent about using the pain medication the surgeon provided. Happily, things have greatly changed. Now you are given nonsteroidal anti-inflammatory drops and pills before and after surgery to prevent pain. Only one in approximately 10 persons need a pain pill or two after surgery, no more. Celluvisc™, a thick artificial tear, helps to relieve the foreign body sensation.

2. *Is radial keratotomy done with a laser?*
   No. Currently, true RK is performed using a very fine, sharp diamond blade knife. There are, however, a number of ongoing FDA-approved studies evaluating the excimer and holmium lasers as tools to correct refraction errors.

3. *Is radial keratotomy a completely safe surgical procedure?*
   No, because there is no such thing as a "completely safe surgical procedure." In the case of RK surgery, the risks of serious problems developing are low. (You are at a greater risk of danger every time you drive on a freeway.)

Glaucoma Surgery

1. *Has my open-angle or closed-angle glaucoma been cured by surgery and my eyesight restored?*
   No. Unhappily, this is never fully achieved. The surgery will stop the deterioration glaucoma was causing to your eyesight, but it will not allow you to recover what has been lost prior to surgery.

2. *If the surgery for glaucoma was so successful, why do I have to keep taking these medications?*
   The surgery lowered your intraocular pressure and arrested the deterioration temporarily, but the surgery may not achieve a low enough intraocular pressure to be safe. Your eyesight can keep deteriorating if you do not reinforce the effect of the surgery on a continuing basis to avoid or forestall the need for surgery again at a future date.

   Questions you should ask to familiarize yourself with eye surgery and your ophthalmic surgeon:

   1. *How many years of experience do you have?*
   2. *What are the other choices of treatment available to me? What are the advantages and disadvantages of each?*
   3. *Are you Board Certified?*
   4. *Have you had the special post-graduate courses in the newer methods of (a) cataract surgery, (b) corneal refractive surgery, (c) etc.?*
   5. *How many operations of the types mentioned above have you performed?*
   6. *How many of these surgeries do you perform per year, month, week?*
   7. *What are the most frequent complications you have seen?*
   8. *How frequent are these complications?*
   9. *Is there anything about my case which would increase the chances of complications?*
   10. *What are the chances that complications can be corrected?*
   11. *Is there an additional charge or cost, and if so, how much approximately?*

   Answers obviously will vary, but these questions are sound.

Billing, Fees, and Insurance

1. *Why did I get a personal bill in the mail? I thought Medicare would take care of everything.*
   Medicare pays 80 percent of the *approved* amount of the cost of the surgery or examination. You are responsible for the remaining 20 percent. If your eye doctor accepts Medicare assignment, this means that the difference between what your doctor charged and what Medicare approved will be "written off." For example, say your doctor charged $2,300 for a procedure and Medicare approved $1,500. If your doctor accepts Medicare assignment, the $800 difference is "written off" and you will never be charged for it. Say Medicare approved this $1,500 but only paid $1,200. The $300 difference between what Medicare approved and actually paid is the 20 percent that you are responsible for. You are always responsible for the 20 percent (the difference between what Medicare approves and what Medicare actually pays) whether the doctor accepts Medicare assignment or not. If your doctor does not accept Medicare assignment, you are responsible for the difference between what your doctor charges and Medicare approves ($800) plus your 20 percent ($300).

2. *Why, after surgery, am I getting bills for professional services from people other than my ophthalmologist?*
   If the surgery was done at a typical out-patient surgical center or hospital, there are separate fees for the use of different facilities. Also, one of the bills most likely is from the anesthesiologist, who assisted the surgeon but has no financial interrelationship with him, the center, or the hospital. Other sources of bills may be laboratory clinical fees, EKG fees, cardiologist charges, and charges from the pathologist who evaluated the excised tissue.

3. *I can't afford to pay the entire difference between the total expenses of the surgery I need and what Medicare will allow. What can I do? I need the surgery badly.?*
   Unfortunately, the government has been reducing the extent to which Medicare provides funds for surgery. Most ophthalmological clinics will work out a credit arrangement with you.

You can pay on a monthly or quarterly basis at a feasible level so you won't have to defer necessary surgical help.

4. *What is Co-Management?*
Co-Management is becoming more and more prevalent in ophthalmology. This is where your eyecare is shared by your operating ophthalmologist, and a skilled optometrist. After the ophthalmologist has performed your surgical procedure, you receive your follow-up care by an optometrist, who then monitors you on a regular basis throughout your healing process. Generally, your ophthalmologist formats a criteria of management guidelines for various surgical procedures. Communication lines are always open between your ophthalmologist and your optometrist concerning your eyecare during recovery. Once you are ready for a new pair of glasses, the optometrist fits them accordingly.

Miscellaneous Questions

1. *What is the difference between an ophthalmologist, an optometrist and an optician?*
An *ophthalmologist* is a medical doctor specializing in medical and surgical treatment of eye diseases and disorders. After completion of medical school, the ophthalmologist completes a "residency" which is approximately a three- to five-year further intensive study of the eye. The ophthalmologist is licensed to diagnose conditions, treat medical conditions either by performing surgery or prescribing medications, and to prescribe and dispense contact lenses or eyeglasses.

An *optometrist* completes four years of optometry school after completion of four years of undergraduate studies and is referred to as a "doctor of optometry" or O.D. The optometrist is qualified to detect many eye disorders, such as infection, a foreign body, previous trauma, glaucoma, retinal problems, and cataracts, but is not a medical doctor. An optometrist's primary function is to determine eye characteristics, and to prescribe and dispense eyeglasses and contact lenses. In various states, the optometrist is licensed to treat certain medical problems and to provide co-management with an ophthalmologist.

An *optician* is an artisan who grinds and fits prescribed lenses. An optician is skilled in the cosmetic and functional selection of eyeglass frames and lenses with various features and characteristics.

2. *To read I have to hold text out away from me, and my arms are getting too short! Can anything be done to help?*
   Yes. We have been involved in the early preliminary evaluation of this condition, and the study of the Schachar Presbyopia Band, the latest surgical technique to correct presbyopia. Initial results have returned near visual ability to about six inches, with the ability to read the telephone book print.

3. *I can't read anymore. Are "drug store readers" going to hurt my eyes?*
   No. The over-the-counter reading glasses are helpful if all you need is magnification. They work well if the vision in both eyes is equal and no significant astigmatism is present.

4. *When I look at my prescriptions, what do the abbreviations mean?*

o.u.	= both eyes	o.d.	= right eye
o.s.	= left eye	P.O.	= by mouth
p.r.n.	= as needed	q	= every
R.E.	= right eye	q.d.	= once daily
L.E.	= left eye	h.s.	= bedtime
b.i.d.	= two times daily	q.o.d.	= every other day
t.i.d.	= three times daily	q.4.d.	= every four days
q4h	= every four hours	ml.	= milliliter
A.C.	= before you eat	mg.	= milligram
P.C.	= after you eat	gtt.	= drop
q.h.s.	= every time at bedtime	ung.	= ointment
oph.sol.	= ophthalmic solution		
oph.ung	= ophthalmic ointment		

5. *I see well, do I have to drive with glasses on?*
   The answer in most states is clear and specific. If you see 20/40 or worse in one or both eyes without correction, and you can be corrected by glasses and/or contact lenses to see better than 20/40, you are required to wear correction. For example, if you

are 20/20 R.E. and 20/50 L.E., and, if by wearing correction for your L.E., you will see better, you must wear correction. Conversely, if the left eye is a "lazy eye," or amblyopic, and no glasses will make it better, then if the doctor certifies you, no restriction about wearing glasses is placed on your driver's license.

6. *How do I put my drops in my eyes?*
The proper way to put a drop into the eye is to pull the lower outer eyelid forward and down gently a little bit to form a "cup" into which the drop may be placed. Normal blinking will then distribute the liquid onto the eye surface.

If you wish to minimize systemic absorption of the eyedrop, as may be the case with beta-blockers, after instilling the eyedrop, close your eyes then gently press your index fingers into the corners (toward the nose) of your eyes. This will block the punctum and will decrease eyedrop drainage into the nose and throat.

7. *Do dilating eyedrops affect my blood pressure?*
Yes they can. A word of caution. If you have severe hypertension, and have arteriosclerotic heart disease with arrythmia, tell the technician who is responsible for the dilation of your eyes. Neosynephrine 10 percent is sometimes used to dilate the eyes and may elevate your blood pressure. The Neosynephrine 2.5 percent or other eyedrops might be safer.

8. *Can I put two different types of eyedrops in my eye at the same time?*
The answer is yes, but you may lose much of the drug effect. The eye can only hold two single drops at a time. Any excess merely runs out. We generally advise a minimum wait of five minutes between different types of eyedrops. A better idea is to use one type before you eat and the other type after you eat.

9. *Does using my roommate's prescription eye medications for the same kind of problem hurt my eyes?*
Self-diagnosis can be dangerous. Many similar-looking conditions may actually be very different indeed. Trying to treat yourself could complicate matters, even cause decreased vision or other problems.

10. *I have a lot of drops left after my last infection. What should I do with them?*

    First, unless otherwise indicated on the label, you were supposed to use your drops, pills, or ointment until the prescription was finished. Your chances of recovering from an eye condition by using leftover, half-full bottles is problematic at best.

11. *What are floaters?*

    The older Latin term for vitreous floaters may help you understand their nature. The Latin term for vitreous floaters is *muscae volitantes* meaning "fluttering flies." Floaters are usually the result of normal aging changes in the eye, but may occasionally signal serious internal eye problems. When you are young, the vitreous cavity is filled with a very thick, sticky gel containing many very small collagen microfibrils. As you mature, the gel changes to a liquid. This process is called *syneresis.* The gel in the vitreous does not melt like gelatin, rather it develops pockets of water similar to Swiss cheese. These pockets are generally in the center of the gel ball and around the outside over areas of abnormal retina. The particles, formerly in the gel, are now suspended in liquid and clump together into slightly opaque forms of varying shapes similar to "mosquitos," "spots," "cobwebs," "rings," "serpents," etc. The heavier, denser gel eventually peels away from the inside of the retina, collapsing into the synerectic cavities. Quick eye movements then cause a whip-like movement of the gel and its opaque particles to move around inside of the eye.

12. *Are vitreous floaters dangerous?*

    The sudden appearance of floaters is frequently preceded by flashes of light when traction of the vitreous "pulls" on the retina. If the gel peels off without tearing a hole, no damage has been done. If the gel adheres tightly to the retina, the collapse may be associated with pulling a hole in the retina. If this happens, you must have it repaired. Floaters may also be pigmented cells from the torn retina or red blood cells from torn capillaries in the retina. Immediate treatment by laser or cryotherapy may prevent the need for a scleral buckling procedure.

Other abnormal and dangerous causes of floaters could be blood in the eye caused from diabetic retinopathy, hypertension, neovascularization and other retinal conditions. Hemorrhages in the vitreous body are often seen as clumps, black streaks, or black pepper spots.

Floaters may even be from white blood cells, either single or clumped together as in conditions of iritis and vitritis.

13. *Do I need to be checked for floaters?*
In most instances get an eye exam when convenient. If the floaters are black and you see flashes of light whenever you move your eye, matters could be urgent and you should see your ophthalmologist immediately.

14. *What is ophthalmic migraine?*
Ophthalmic migraine is a variety of the common migraine headache in which the patient feels no immediate pain but may see a variety of different visual disturbances. Ophthalmic migraine generally starts with a jagged "running W" in the peripheral visual area. This may progress to blurring of vision. Other examples are: loss of central vision, loss of peripheral vision with central vision spared, loss of vision on the right side or left side, progressive loss of color vision similar to your color television slowly changing to black and white, and irregular blurring such as looking through a window pane with water running down the surface.

These visual abnormalities usually last about 12 to 20 minutes but may last several hours. They are usually progressive and typically disappear almost instantly. Usually you have only a minor headache, if any, afterward. Patients generally have a strong family history of migraine headaches. Contributing factors may be foods, hormones, especially early in premenstrual cycles, flashes of light and stress. One characteristic of ophthalmic migraine is that you see the disturbance in both eyes whether the eyes are open or closed.

15. *What is a migraine headache?*
    This is a specific type of headache best treated by your personal physician or neurologist. There is generally a strong family history of such headaches and females are more commonly afflicted than males. Migraines generally start between age 15 and 30 and may be exacerbated by birth control pills and after years of dormancy may reoccur about the age of 60.

    Initially, the blood vessels go into spasm causing prodromal symptoms of visual flashes or scintillating blind spots, drowsiness, and peripheral numbness in the legs and arms. Vasodilation of vessels follows with the associated, usually severe, headache, nausea, vomiting, and light sensitivity. Avoiding certain foods is wise in migraine headaches. They are: chocolate, anything pickled, broad beans (pinto, navy, lima), nuts, figs, raisins, avocados, ripe bananas, chicken livers, chipped beef, sausage, salami, pepperoni, hot dogs, yeast breads, soy sauce, cheeses (especially aged or cottage), milk, sour cream, ice cream, cream, yogurt, butter (corn oil is okay), red wine vinegar or salad dressing, most alcohol, especially wine and beer (scotch and brandy are generally okay), caffeine and caffeine-containing cola beverages. See your personal physician regarding treatment.

16. *What is temporomandibular joint pain?*
    Temporomandibular joint (TMJ) pain is one of the most common causes of headache seen by the eye care specialist. The TMJ is the large joint that allows the lower jaw to open and close. You may have pain in the temples if you press the area. Because of its proximity to the eyes, you may think the eyes are causing the pain. TMJ pain is associated with a jaw that "clicks" when opened wide, or when teeth position is poor such as in overbite, underbite, uneven teeth after braces, shifting or tooth movement due to impacted wisdom teeth, and tooth extractions. Individuals with all the teeth removed may experience atrophy of the gum mucosa under the false teeth, which may cause progressive, excessive closure or movement of the lower jaw.

Bitemporal pain is frequently present upon awakening, due to grinding the teeth while sleeping. The pain may develop and increase during work hours if you have a high-stress job because you "lock your teeth down" and maintain excessive pressures on your back teeth. Stressful periods in our lives are often accompanied by these pains.

Many dentists and oral surgeons, orthodontists, and ENT specialists are trained to evaluate and correct these problems.

17. *I frequently have styes. Can I use a special soap to prevent them?*
Yes. In our clinic, we studied patients with severe styes, meibomitis, and corneal ulcers such that they required antibiotic eyedrops, ointment, oral antibiotics, and hot compresses. Out of the 287 cases, 89 percent were using non-deodorant soaps. The most common soaps among infected patients were Ivory™ (59 percent), Dove™ (20 percent), Neutrogena™ (10 percent). The balance of the cases used any number of different soaps or only water. Only 11 percent of the patients used deodorant soaps such as Dial™, Safeguard™, and Irish Spring™. Of note is that Ivory™ soap represents approximately 8 percent of sales in our market, and deodorant soaps represent approximately 70 percent of our market.

Wrap-Up

- A comprehensive eye examination takes about two hours and usually will entail dilation of your eyes. Dilation lasts approximately 30 minutes to four hours and will cause light sensitivity. It is wise to bring someone with you to the doctor's office to drive you back home or to work.
- Vasoconstrictor eyedrops, such as Visine™ for "red eyes" should be used sparingly once or twice a month.
- A cataract is an opacity of the natural crystalline lens. It cannot be scraped off or removed with a laser. It must be surgically removed.
- Cataract surgery is painless.

- Recovery from cataract surgery is remarkably fast. Generally, no hospital stay is necessary and you can return to work the following day. However, you should abstain from heavy lifting and strenuous activity for at least three weeks following surgery.
- Vision following cataract surgery may fluctuate for a couple of weeks. Thereafter, vision is usually clear and colors are bright. If necessary, eyeglasses or contact lenses may be prescribed one to two months following surgery.
- Radial keratotomy (RK) is a painless surgical procedure designed to reduce or eliminate nearsightedness. RK involves making incisions in the cornea which alter the shape of the cornea, thus reducing nearsightedness.
- RK is not performed with a laser at this time, although the excimer and holmium lasers are currently under FDA investigation for the correction of refractive errors.
- There currently is no cure for glaucoma, and visual loss from glaucoma is irreversible. In most cases, glaucoma can be controlled if the prescribed treatment is faithfully adhered to.
- Medicare pays 80 percent of the approved amount of your surgery. You are responsible for the remaining 20 percent. Often, patients have a supplemental insurance company which pays the remaining 20 percent.
- It is very important that you find out if your eye doctor accepts Medicare assignment. If he does not, you may be responsible for expenses that you are not prepared for. Discuss your financial obligations with your doctor's insurance department.
- If you are about 40 years of age or more and have discovered that you are no longer able to read because "your arms are too short," you probably have presbyopia. Presbyopia is a normal process and is easily corrected with reading glasses.
- Never use another person's eye medications or use old medications.

- Most floaters are harmless and appear as gray spots or fluttering flies, but should be checked promptly by your eye doctor. Symptoms which should be checked immediately are seeing flashes of light and/or hundreds of black floaters.
- Ophthalmic migraine causes a variety of temporary visual disturbances whether the eyes are open or closed. Symptoms include seeing a jagged "running W" in your peripheral visual area, loss of central vision, loss of color vision, and irregular blurring. Ophthalmic migraines usually do not cause a headache.
- Temporomandibular joint (™J) pain is a common cause of headache. The TMJ is the joint that allows the jaw to open and close.
- The use of deodorant soaps has been shown to effectively reduce the occurrence of styes, meibomitis, and corneal ulcers if used on a regular basis.

Bibliography

Abrams, D., *Ophthalmology in Medicine*, C. V. Mosby, St. Louis, 1990.

Abrams, W. B. and R. Berkow, *Merck Manual of Geriatrics*, Merck, Sharp, Dohme Research Laboratories, Archway, NJ, 1990.

Albert, Daniel M. and Frederick A. Jakobiec, *Principles and Practice of Ophthalmology: Clinical Practice*, Vol. I, W. B. Saunders Co., Philadelphia, 1994.

Buck, *Physiological Zoolology*, University of Chicago Press, Chicago, Vol. 10, p. 412, 1937.

Callahan, Alston, *Reconstructive Surgery of the Eyelids and Ocular Adnexa*, Aesculpapius Publishing, Birmingham, Ala., 1966.

Cohen, N. S. and J. I. Schapiro, *Out of Vision Into Sight*, Simon & Schuster, New York, 1977.

Crabb, J. L., *I Can See*, Peachtree Publishers, Ltd., Memphis, 1988.

Crater, John, *Sudden Vision*, Slack, Inc. Thorofare, NJ, 1990.

Duke-Elder, Sir Stewart, *System of Ophthalmology*, Vol. I, *The Eye In Evolution*, Kimpton, London, 1958.

———, *The Practice of Refraction*, 7th Ed., C. V. Mosby, St. Louis, 1965.

———, and Arthur George Leigh, *System of Ophthalmology*, Vol. VIII, *Diseases of the Outer Eye*, Part 2, *Cornea and Sclera*, C. V. Mosby, St. Louis, 1965.

———, and Edward S. Perkins, *System of Ophthalmology*, Vol. IX, *Diseases of the Uveal Tract*, C. V. Mosby, St. Louis, 1966.

———, and Barrie Jay, *System of Ophthalmology*, Vol. XI, *Diseases of the Lens and Vitreous; Glaucoma and Hypotony*, C. V. Mosby, St. Louis, 1969.

Fronterre, A. and G. P. Portesani, *Refractive and Corneal Surgery,* Vol. 7, No. 2, 1991, "Comparison of Epikeratophakia and Penetrating Keratoplasty for Keratoconus," pp. 167-173.

Gills, James P., *Wonderful Glorious Sight,* Cataract and Intraocular Lens Institute, Tarpon Springs, 1988.

Gilman, Alfred Goodman, et al., *The Pharmacological Basis of Therapeutics,* 8th ed., McGraw-Hill, 1990.

Goldberg, Stephen, *Ophthalmology Made Ridiculously Simple,* Medmaster, Miami, 1982.

Gorin, George, *History of Ophthalmology,* Publish or Perish, Wilmington, Del., 1982.

Harrington, D. V., *The Visual Fields,* C. V. Mosby Co., St. Louis, 1964.

Hartline, Wagner and MacNichol, *Cold Spring Harbor Symposia on Quantitative Biology,* 1952, Cold Spring Harbor Laboratory, Cold Spring, New York, Vol. 17, p. 125.

Henkes, H. E. and C. L. Zrennas, *History of Ophthalmology,* Kluwer Academic Publishers, Dordrecht, Holland, 1988.

Jenner, *Anatomical Records III,* A. R. Liss, New York, 1952, p. 512.

Kavner, R. S. and L. Dusky, *Total Vision,* A & W Publishers, New York, 1938.

Kelman, Charles D., *Through My Eyes,* Cross Publishers, New York, 1985.

March, Wayne F., *Practical Ophthalmic Problems,* Warren H. Green, St. Louis, 1986.

Minchin, *Proceeding Royal Society B 60,* Royal Society of London, 1986, p. 42.

Moore, C. R., *VIP Syndrome—Evaluation and Medical Management,* Proc. Sixth Biennial Cataract Surgical Congress, C. V. Mosby Co., St. Louis, 1980.

———, *Comparison of Extra Capsular and Intra Capsular IOL Procedures,* Proc. Sixth Biennial Cataract Surgical Congress, C. V. Mosby Co., St. Louis, 1980.

Moses, Robert A., *Adler's Physiology of the Eye: Clinical Application,* C. V. Mosby Co., St. Louis, 1970.

Neal, Helen, *Low Vision,* Simon & Schuster, New York, 1987.

Newell, F. W., *Ophthalmology Principles and Concepts,* C. V. Mosby Co., St. Louis, 1969.

Parks, Marshall M., *Ocular Motility and Strabismus,* Harper and Row, New York, 1975.

Rubman, R. H. and H. Rothman, *Future Vision*, Dodd, Mead, New York, 1957.

Sanders, D. R. and R. P. Hoffman, *Refractive Surgery, A Text of Radial Keratotomy*, Slack, Inc., Thorofare, NJ, 1985.

────── and R. P. Hoffman, and J. J. Salz, *Corneal Refractive Surgery*, Slack, Inc., Thorofare, NJ, 1985.

Schwab, I. R., *Refractive Keratoplasty*, Churchill Livingston, New York, 1987.

Seiderman, A. S. and S. E. Marcus, *20/20 Is Not Enough*, Alfred A. Knopf, New York, 1989.

Shingleton, B. J., P. S. Hersh and K. R. Kenyou, *Eye Trauma*, Mosby-Year Book, Inc., St. Louis, 1991.

Shulman, Julius, *Cataracts*, Scott, Foresman, Washington D. C., 1984.

──────, *No More Glasses*, Simon & Schuster, New York, 1987.

Sloane, Albert E., *So You Have Cataracts*, Charles C. Thomas, Springfield, 1975.

Vaughn, D., A. Taylor and K. F. Tabbars, *General Ophthalmology*, Appleton and Lange, Norwalk, 1989.

Veirs, E. R., *So You Have Glaucoma*, 2nd ed., Grune and Stratton, New York, 1970.

Wolff, E. and R. J. Last, *Anatomy of the Eye and Orbit*, W. B. Saunders Co., Philadelphia, 1968.

Winograd, L. A. and M. L. Rubin, *Triad Eye Care Notes*, Triad Publishing Co., Gainesville, 1990.

Zinn, W. J. and H. Soloman, *Complete Guide to Eye Care, Eye Glasses, and Contact Lenses*, Frederich Fell, Hollywood, FL, 1986.

Index

absolute hyperopia, 66
accommodation, 28, 58, 59
accommodative convergence, 66
Acquired Immune Deficiency
    Syndrome (AIDS), 140, 265
acute-angle closure glaucoma
    (CAG), 98, 104
acute congestive glaucoma, 98, 104
age-related macular degeneration
    (ARMD), 130–34
aging process
    and cataract formation, 29, 73–74
    and central serous retinopathy,
        137–38
    and contact lens use, 110–11
    and cosmetic surgery, 12–13,
        243–47
    floaters in, 28, 43, 45, 259–60,
        288–89
    loss of endothelial cells in, 21,
        50–51
    presbyopia in, 28–29, 116, 194,
        220–21, 286
    and radial keratotomy, 117
    tear production and, 23, 242
    vitreous detachment in, 45
"air puff" tonometers, 44
alcohol, 74, 145, 251
Alhazen, 5
allergic conjunctivitis, 163
allergies, 37
allowances, insurance, 270
alternate cover test, 37
alternating strabismus, 150
amblyopia ("lazy eye"), 150, 219–20
Amsler grid test, 51
anatomy of the eye, 15–33
    angle/trabecular meshwork, 26

anterior chamber, 17–18, 25
aqueous humor, 18, 26
ciliary body, 27
conjunctiva, 19, 24
cornea, 16, 18–21
crystalline lens, 28–29
early awareness of, 4–6, 9
general description, 16–18
iris, 26–27
lids and tears, 21–23
posterior chamber, 18, 26
pupil, 26
retina, 30–32
sclera, 16–17, 19, 25
vitreous cavity, 18, 27–28
ancient period, 1–2
angle, 18
angle of refraction, 61
angle-recession glaucoma, 99
angle/trabecular meshwork,
    anatomy of, 26
anisometropia, 58, 219–20,
    228–29
anterior, as term, 15
anterior chamber
    anatomy of, 17–18, 25
    fundus photographs of, 50
anterior epithelium basement
    membrane dystrophy, 166
anterior uveitis, 168
antioxidants, 74
antiseptics, 9
aphakia, 66, 219
applanation tonometry, 44
aqueous, 19
aqueous humor
    anatomy of, 18, 26
    early awareness of, 4, 6

aqueous humor *(cont.)*
  in glaucoma, 96
  loss of, treatment for, 4
Arab countries, 5, 6
argon laser trabeculoplasty (ALT), 88–89, 101–3
arthritis, 265
artificial tears, 23, 173, 242
assignment, insurance, 270
astigmatism, 58, 69, 118, 119, 194
  in children, 152
  and contact lenses, 214, 220
  correction of, 6
  determining degree of, 41–42
  lenses for, 65
  physiology of, 17
atheromatous vascular plaques, 260
autoimmune disease, 23, 260, 265
automated lamellar keratectomy or keratoplasty (ALK), 119, 122–23
automatic refractors, 40–41
avascular, 19

Babylonian empire, 1
background diabetic retinopathy, 135
Bacon, Roger, 6
bandage soft contact lenses (BSCL), 221–22
Barroquer, Jose, 122
basal cell carcinoma, 241
Bausch & Lomb, 217
benefits, insurance, 270
bifocal lenses, 29, 69, 70–71, 196, 205
  contact lenses, 221
  development of, 6, 9
  progressive, 71, 196, 198, 205
  types of, 197–99
  vision examination for, 40
black eyes (shiners), 261
black floaters, 45, 259–60, 289
blepharitis, 158–59, 161, 172

blepharoplasty (eyelid lift), 13, 244–47
blindness
  from age-related macular degeneration, 131
  congenital, 146
  due to blood problems, 260
  hysterical, 264
  legal, 38
blind spots, 48, 134, 137
  in glaucoma, 95
blinking, 21–23
blow out fractures, 261
blurred vision (ametropia), 57
Bowman's membrane, 19
branch retinal vein occlusion, 46–47
brunescence, 74
bullae (blisters), 168, 170
buphthalmos ("ox eye"), 99, 148
Bush, Barbara, 238

canaliculi ducts, 23
canaliculitis, 174
cancer, 86
  of the eyelid, 240–41
  see also tumors
carriers, insurance, 269–70, 271
cataracts, 73–84
  as cause of glaucoma, 99
  congenital, 74, 146, 147
  contrast sensitivity examination for, 51
  corneal degeneration from, 182
  formation of, 29, 73–74
  lenses for, 70
  prevention of, 74
  secondary, 74, 79, 91
  surgery for. *see* cataract surgery
  symptoms of, 43, 45
  types of, 74
cataract surgery, 8
  common questions, 281–82
  "couching," 2, 3
  cryosurgical extraction, 75–76

early use of, 2, 3
extracapsular extraction, 76
intracapsular extraction, 74–75
intraocular lens implant (IOL) in, 29, 73, 76, 80, 112–13, 147
lasers in, 79–80
loss of endothelial cells in, 21
operating procedures for, 80–83
phacoemulsification, 76–78
polymethylmethacrylate (PMMA) lenses, 13, 216
removal of cataract, 9, 74–83
success of, 82–83
cellophane retinopathy, 137
Celsus, 3, 4
central retinal artery occlusion, 46–47
central serous retinopathy, 137–38
central vision, 51–52
cerebral stroke, 264
chalazions, 159–60
Champus insurance, 273
chemical hazards, 262
children. *see* pediatric eye care
chlamydial infection, 146
choroidal neovascular membrane (CNVM), 130–34
choroidal nevus, 141
choroidal rupture, 133–34
chromatic aberration, 58–59
chronic open-angle glaucoma (COAG), 95–96, 99–104
ciliary body, anatomy of, 27
classical period, 2–4
clear lensectomy, 113
cocaine, 251, 252
Cogan's microcystic dystrophy, 166
co-insurance, 271
color bodies, 26–27
colored contact lenses, 219
color vision examination, 51–52
co-management, 82, 285
computerized corneal topographer (CCT), 53–54
concave lenses, 64, 65

cones, 30, 51
congenital disorders
blindness, 146
cataracts, 74, 146, 147
glaucoma, 99, 104–5, 147–48
conjunctiva
anatomy of, 19, 24
infections of, 8, 9, 24, 42, 146, 163–64
tears and, 23
conjunctivitis. *see* pinkeye
contact lenses, 71, 213–31
and aging process, 110–11, 221
and anisometropia, 228–29
and astigmatism, 214, 220
bandage soft contact lenses (BSCL), 221–22
for children, 153, 219–20
colored, 219
costs of, 217–18
decision to wear, 229–30
described, 213–15
disposable, 202, 218
driving with, 287
evolution of, 215–19
extended-wear, 201, 202, 218
eyeglasses versus, 201–2
fitting and adaptation, 222–24
hard, 202, 216
infections and complications from, 224–27
and orthokeratology, 227–28
and presbyopia, 220–21
and progress of myopia, 67
prosthetic, 222
refraction with, 38
and refractometry, 40–42
rigid gas-permeable (RGP), 202, 215, 217, 219, 222–23, 227–28
soft, 201–2, 215–19, 223–27
tinted, 218–19
contrast sensitivity examination, 51
convergence, and drug use, 255
convergent strabismus, 66, 149–50

convex lenses, 64, 65
cornea
    anatomy of, 16, 18–21
    astigmatism. *see* astigmatism
    early awareness of, 5
    edema of, 167–69, 182, 216, 217
    in external and front chamber eye examination, 42
    fundus photographs of, 50
    herpetic infections, 176–78
    injuries to, 164–65
    keratoconus, 42, 68, 117, 178, 182, 227
    keratoplasty, 9–10
    pinguecuela, 180–81
    pterygium, 179–80
    tears and, 23
    transplants of, 9–12, 115, 121, 126, 169–70, 178, 181–83, 227
    ulcers, 1, 170–72, 225
corneal diseases, 8
corneal dystrophies, 165–66
corneal endothelial cell count, 50–51
corneal filtrates, 225–26
corneal guttata, 167
corneal hypoxia, 225
corneal refractive surgery, 10–12, 90–91, 113–27
    automated lamellar keratoplasty, 119, 122–23
    epikeratophakia, 12, 115, 122, 124–25, 147
    excimer laser, 120–21
    hyperopic hexagonal keratotomy, 127
    keratomileusis, 11, 12, 115, 122
    keratophakia, 11, 115, 125
    penetrating keratoplasty (corneal transplant), 9–12, 115, 121, 126, 169–70, 178, 181–83, 227
    radial keratotomy. *see* radial keratotomy (RK)
    refractive corneal keratectomy, 125–26
    refractive keratoplasty, 10–12, 121–22
    Ruiz procedure, 127
    thermokeratoplasty, 115, 126–27
corneal topography analysis, 178
corneal vascularization, 225
corneo-scleral contact lenses, 215
cosmetic surgery, 12–13, 243–47
"couching," 2, 3
covered expenses, insurance, 271
crossed eyes, 9, 50, 66, 148–55
cryolathe, 11, 12
cryopexy, 139
cryosurgical extraction, 75–76
crystalline lens
    anatomy of, 28–29
    and cataracts, 45
    fundus photographs of, 50
cyclocryotherapy, 101
cycloplegic agents, 165
cystoid macular edema (CME), 76
cytomegalovirus (CMV), 140, 265

dacryocystitis, 174
dacryocystorhinostomy (DCR), 174
"dancing eyes" (nystagmus), 146, 255
deductible, insurance, 271, 273
dellen, 179
Democritus, 3, 4
dendritic keratitis, 177
depth perception examination, 52–53
dermatochalasis (baggy upper eyelids), 235–37
Descemet's membrane, anatomy of, 20
diabetes, 8–9, 264
    and blockages of veins and arteries, 260
    cataracts from, 74
    as cause of glaucoma, 99

contrast sensitivity examination
  for, 51
and eye examinations, 191
refractive index in, 66
symptoms of, 43, 47, 66
and vitreous hemorrhage, 260
diabetic retinopathy, 9, 47, 134–36
diffraction, of electromagnetic
  radiation, 62
dilated examination, 44–47, 68
  for children, 152
  common questions, 280, 287
  and hypertension, 287
dilator muscles, 27
diopter lenses, 65
diopters, 59
diplopia, 151–52
disposable contact lenses, 202, 218
distance vision, 38
divergent strabismus, 69, 149–50
Down's syndrome, 146
driving
  after cataract surgery, 81
  with dilated eyes, 280
  with glasses or contact lenses,
    286–87
  and glaucoma, 93, 94
drug use, 249–57
  Fetal Alcohol Syndrome (FAS),
    145
  OpticALERTTM test, 250–56
dry eyes, 47–48, 172–73, 242

ectropion (turning-out eyelids),
  172, 239–40
edema
  corneal, 120, 167–69, 182, 216,
    217
  cystoid muscular (CME), 76
  retinal, 135
effective date of policy, 271
Egypt, 2, 6–8
electromagnetic radiation, 60, 62,
  74, 86–88

electroretinogram (ERG), 52
emergencies, ocular, 259–67
  blindness due to blood problems,
    260
  blunt trauma, 260–61, 264
  cerebral stroke, 264
  chemical hazards, 262
  cuts or punctures, 261–62
  hysterical blindness, 264
  metamorphopsia, 264
  optic neuritis, 51, 262–63
  orbital cellulitis, 161, 162, 263
  paracentesis, 9, 101
  retinal detachment, 13, 45, 68,
    138–40, 259–60
  rubeosis, 43, 265
  ultraviolet light injuries, 87,
    263–64
  uveitis, 99, 105, 265–66
emmetropia, 38, 57, 118
endophotocoagulation, 136
endophthalmitis infection, 120
endothelium, 26
  anatomy of, 20–21
  corneal endothelial cell count,
    50–51
  hereditary diseases of, 167
  injuries to, 166
  loss of, 21, 50–51, 167–68
  perforation of, 120, 167
entropion (turning in eyelids), 172,
  238–39
enucleation, 141, 266
epikeratophakia, 12, 115, 122,
  124–25, 147
epiphora, 173–74
episcleritis, 174–75
epithelium
  anatomy of, 19
  erosion of, 120
  injuries to, 166
  loss of, 87
equator, 15
erosion, of cornea, 165
esotropia, 149–50

"evil eye," 3
evisceration, 141, 243, 266
excessive tearing, 173–74, 241–43
excimer laser, 90–91, 120–21
exclusions, insurance, 271
exophthalmometry examination, 49
exotropia, 149–50
explanation of benefits (E.O.B.), 271–72
extended-wear contact lenses, 201, 202, 218
external and front chamber eye examination, 42–43
external hordeolum, 159
external photographs, 50
extracapsular extraction, 76
eyeball, removal of, 141, 243, 266
eyebrows, drooping (eyebrow ptosis), 235
eye care
 in ancient and classical periods, 1–4
 in the early modern period, 6–9
 in the Middle Ages, 4–6
 in the modern period, 10–13
eye chart, 38, 40
eyedrops
 applying, 287
 common questions, 280–81, 287–88
 for dilated examination, 45, 280, 287
eye examinations, 35–55
 allergies and, 37
 chief complaint in, 36
 common questions, 278–80
 medical and eye history in, 36, 190
 medications and, 37
 routine tests, 37–47, 190–91
 special tests, 47–54
eyeglasses, 9, 187–211
 after cataract surgery, 82
 for children, 152–53
 contact lenses versus, 201–2
 costs of, 191–93
 driving with, 286–87
 early use of, 6
 examinations for, 37–47, 189–91
 frames, 196–97
 lenses, 69–71, 194–96, 199–201, 205–6. *see also* bifocal lenses; trifocal lenses
 materials for, 199–201
 problems with, 204–6
 purposes of, 194–98
 and refractometry, 40–42
 suppliers of, 203–4, 206–11
 waiting for, 193–94
eye history, 36, 190
eyelid ptosis (drooping eyelids), 234–35
eyelid retraction, 237–38
eyelids, 234–41
 after cataract surgery, 82
 anatomy of, 21–23
 corrective surgery for, 234–40
 cosmetic surgery for, 13, 243–47
 infections of, 158–62
 lower, laxity of, 238–39
 lower, lift of (blepharoplasty), 13, 245, 246
 staring, 237–38, 252
 turning in (entropion), 238–39
 turning out (ectropion), 239–40
 upper, baggy (dermatochalasis), 235–37
 upper, drooping, 234–35, 252
 upper, lift of (blepharoplasty), 244–46
eye muscle examination, 37
eye muscles, 16
 dilator, 27
 imbalances in, 37, 66, 69, 148–55, 219
 sphincter, 27
eye shields, 80–82
eye tracking, and drug use, 254–55

Farnsworth color disks, 52
farsightedness (hyperopia), 57, 65–66, 118, 194
 in children, 152–53

early treatment of, 3–4
epikeratophakia for, 12
physiology of, 17
plus lenses for, 17
Fetal Alcohol Syndrome (FAS), 145
field test, 48, 49, 95, 191
flat-top bifocals, 197
floaters
  black, 45, 259–60, 289
  gray, 28, 43, 45, 259–60, 288–89
fluid attractional force, 213
fluorescein angiography, 49–50, 131, 132, 133
focal macular photocoagulation, 135
fornix, 24
fovea, 30, 129–30
frames, eyeglass, 196–97
Franklin, Benjamin, 6, 9
Franklin bifocals, 198
Fuchs' dystrophy, 166, 167
fundus photographs, 50
fusion, 150

Galen, 3, 4
gamma globulins, 23
Gaylord, Norman, 217
geniculate bodies, 30
geometric axis, 15
Giant Papillary Conjunctivitis (GPC), 226–27
Gills, James, 82–83
glands of Moll, 158–59
glands of Zeis, 158–59
glasses. *see* eyeglasses
glaucoma, 93–107
  acute-angle closure (CAG), 98, 104
  chronic open-angle (COAG), 95–96, 99–104
  congenital, 99, 104–5, 147–48
  diagnosing, 93–95
  early treatment of, 3
  and eye examinations, 191
  gonioscopy examination for, 48, 105

  infantile, 147–48
  and intraocular pressure measurement, 43–44, 94–95, 190
  laser surgery for, 13, 88–89, 101–4
  loss of endothelial cells in, 21
  low-tension, 96–98
  medications for, 100–103
  and myopia, 68
  nature of, 93
  rainbow effect in, 62
  secondary, 99, 105, 120, 260
  surgery for, 9, 101–6, 283
  symptoms of, 43, 46, 50, 93–95
  traumatic, 99, 260
  visual field test for, 48, 49, 95, 191
glaucoma suspect, 94–95
Goldman Visual Field Test, 48, 49
gonio lens, 95
gonioscopy examination, 48, 105
Goosey, John, 124–25
gradient lenses, 71
grafts, corneal, 9–12
Graves' disease, 237–38
gray floaters, 28, 43, 45, 259–60, 288–89
Greece, ancient, 3–4
group health insurance, 272–73

hard contact lenses, 202, 216
hard exudates, 135
headaches, 36, 70, 264
  migraine, 289–90
  temporomandibular joint (TMJ), 290–91
Health Maintenance Organization (HMO), 276
heroin, 251, 252
herpes simplex, 168, 176–78
herpes zoster, 168, 176
herpetic infections, 176–78
high myopia, 113, 134
Hippocrates, 3, 4

histoplasmosis, 133–34
HIV, 140
holmium laser thermal keratotomy, 126–27
hyaloid system, 73
hydroxyethylmethacrylate (HEMA), 216
hyperopia. *see* farsightedness (hyperopia)
hyperopic hexagonal keratotomy, 127
hypertension, 260, 264
 and dilated examination, 287
 symptoms of, 46
hyphema, 260
hysterical blindness, 264

Independent Provider Associations/Organizations (IPA/IPO), 277
India, 2
infants. *see* pediatric eye care
infections
 chlamydial, 146
 from contact lens use, 224–27
 eyelid, 158–62
 herpetic, 176–78
 pinkeye. *see* pinkeye (conjunctivitis)
 venereal, 7, 8
inferior, as term, 15
insurance, 269–78
 common questions, 284–85
 group health, 272–73
 Health Maintenance Organizations (HMO), 276
 Independent Provider Associations/Organizations (IPA/IPO), 277
 Medicaid, 273–76
 and ophthalmic plastic surgery, 233–43
 Preferred Provider Organization (PPO) plans, 276–77
 terminology, 269–72

intermediate vision, 40
internal hordeolum, 159
intracapsular cataract extraction, 74–75
intracranial pressure, symptoms of, 46
intraocular lens implant (IOL), 29, 73, 76, 80
 with children, 147
 refractive surgery involving, 112–13
intraocular pressure (IOP)
 measurement of, 43–44, 94–95, 190
 and radial keratotomy, 117–18
 see also glaucoma
iridectomy, 104
iridotomy, 104
 laser surgery for, 88, 90
iris
 anatomy of, 26–27
 pigmentation of, 6
 rubeosis, 43, 265
iritis
 cataracts from, 74
 due to syphilis, 8
Ishihara Color Charts, 52

Japan, 11, 114

Kelman, Charles, 75–76, 76
keratoconus, 42, 68, 117, 178, 182, 227
keratometer, 41–42
keratomileusis, 11, 12, 115, 122
keratophakia, 11, 115, 125
keratoplasty, 9–10
krypton laser, 89

lacquer cracks, 134
lacrimal irrigation, 242
lagophthalmos, 172
lamella, 12

Index

lamellar keratoplasty, 10–12, 121–22
lamellar keratotomy (LK), 182–83
laser photocoagulation, 132–33
laser retinopexy, 139
lasers, 85–92
laser surgery, 13
   argon laser in, 88–89, 101–3
   to close tear drain sites, 23
   excimer laser, 90–91, 120–21
   for glaucoma, 13, 88–89, 101–4
   krypton laser in, 89
   for microaneurysms, 135
   to remove cataracts, 79–80
   YAG neodydium, 89–90, 91, 101, 104
laser thermal keratoplasty, 126–27
lattice degeneration, 138–39
"lazy eye" (amblyopia), 150, 219–20
leeching, 8
legal blindness, 38
lenses, corrective, 69–71, 205–6
   grinding, 195–96
   materials for, 199–201
   see also contact lenses; eyeglasses
lenses, ocular
   accommodation, 28, 58, 59
   crystalline, 28–29, 45, 50
   early awareness of, 5, 6
   implants, 13
   shapes of, 63–65
lensmeter, 50
lenticular lenses, 70
lenticules, 12, 122
lesions
   contrast sensitivity examination for, 51
   symptoms of, 50
limbus, 19
   anatomy of, 16–17
lipids, 23
localized corneal edema, 120
locus vacuus (empty space), 4
low-tension glaucoma, 96–98
low vision aids, 65
Luther, Martin, 6
lysosomes, 23

macula, 129–30
   age-related macular degeneration, 130–34
   Amsler grid test for, 51
   anatomy of, 30
   diabetic retinopathy, 9, 47, 134–36
   in dilated examination, 45–46
   laser surgery for, 89
   macular holes, 136–37
   macular pucker, 137
magnification, 65
map-dot-fingerprint dystrophy, 166
marijuana, 118, 251, 252
measles, cataracts from, 74, 147
Medicaid, 273–76
MediCal, 273
medical history, 36, 190
Medicare, 273–76, 284
meibomian glands, 23
membrane peeling, 137
metamorphopsia, 264
microaneurysms, 135
microcysts, 168
microkeratome, 11–12
Middle Ages, 4–6
migraine headaches, 289–90
mikrokeratoplasty, 12
minification, 65
monovision, 117, 221
mucin, 23
multifocal lenses, 70–71
multiple sclerosis, symptoms of, 46
muscles. *see* eye muscles
mydriatics, 45
myopia. *see* nearsightedness (myopia)
myopic degeneration, 134
myopic keratomileusis (MKM), 122

Napoleon Bonaparte, 6–8
nasolacrimal duct, 23, 174
nearsightedness (myopia), 57, 66–69, 194
   in children, 152

nearsightedness (myopia) *(cont.)*
  corneal refractive surgery for. *see* corneal refractive surgery
  early treatment of, 3–4
  epikeratophakia for, 12
  high, 113, 134
  and orthokeratology, 227–28
  physiology of, 17
near vision card, 38–40
neovascularization, 147
neurological problems, visual field examination for, 48
neurotrophic ulcers, 171
night vision
  blindness, 1
  examination for, 51
  and glaucoma, 100
nuclear cataracts, 74
nystagmus (dancing eyes), 146, 255

occipital visual cortex, 129
ocular hypertensives, 94–95
ocular photography, 49–51
ophthalmic maturity, 150
ophthalmic migraines, 289–90
ophthalmic plastic surgery, 233–43
  abnormal tearing, 241–43
  cancers of the eyelid, 240–41
  eyelid correction, 13, 234–40
ophthalmologists, 188, 189–90, 285
ophthalmoscope
  direct, 45
  indirect, 46
opthalmic assistant, 35
opthalmology
  as discrete branch of medical science, 6, 8
  Middle Ages, 5–6
optical cellulitis, 263
OpticALERTTM test, 250–56
optic chiasm, 30
  early awareness of, 4
optic cup, 95
optic foramen, 16–17
opticians, 71, 188, 189, 195, 286

optic nerve, 16, 30
  degeneration of, symptoms of, 46
  in dilated examination, 45–46, 46
  early awareness of, 4, 5
  fundus photographs of, 50
  and pupil examination, 37
optic neuritis, 51, 262–63
optics, 9, 59–65
optometrists, 188, 189, 285
orbit, 16
orbital cellulitis, 161, 162, 263
orthokeratology, 227–28
ovale, 159
over-refraction, 38
"ox eye" (buphthalmos), 99, 148

pachymetry, 117
pan retinal photocoagulation (PRP), 135–36
paracentesis, 9, 101
paralytic strabismus, 150
partial thickness keratoplasty, 121
participating providers, 272
patching, 153, 154–55, 220
pathological myopia, 68
PCP, 251
pediatric eye care, 145–56
  astigmatism, 152
  contact lenses, 153
  contact lenses for children, 219–20
  disorders in newborns, 99, 104–5, 145–48
  eyeglasses, 152–53
  muscle imbalances, 37, 66, 69, 148–55
penetrating keratoplasty (corneal transplant), 9, 12, 115, 121, 126, 169–70, 178, 181–83, 227
peripheral iridectomy, 104
peripheral iridotomy, 104
peripheral vision
  in glaucoma, 94, 95, 96
  measuring, 191

phacoemulsification, 76–78
phoropter, 42
photocoagulation, 88
photons, 86
physics of light, 9
physiology of sight, 129–30
pigmentation, 26–27
pinguecuela, 180–81
pinhole occluders, 38
pinkeye (conjunctivitis), 9, 24, 42, 146, 163–64
  due to gonorrhea, 8
  treatment of, 2, 163–64
  types of, 163
plastic surgery
  cosmetic, 12–13, 243–47
  ophthalmic, 233–43
plus lenses, 17
pneumatic retinopexy, 139
policy provisions, 271
polycarbonate lenses, 200, 206
polymethylmethacrylate (PMMA) lenses, 13, 216
posterior, as term, 15
posterior chamber, anatomy of, 18, 26
posterior subcapsular cataracts, 74
posterior vitreous detachment (PVD), 141
pre-existing conditions, 272
Preferred Provider Organization (PPO) plans, 276–77
premature infants, 146–47
presbyopia, 28–29, 116, 194
  and contact lenses, 220–21
  surgery for, 286
prescriptions, abbreviations on, 286
primary angle closure glaucoma, 98, 104
Primary Care Physician (PCP), 276
primary carrier, insurance, 271
prisms, 61–62, 63–64
progressive hyperopia, 120
progressive lenses, 71, 196, 198, 205
progressive myopia, 68

proliferative diabetic retinopathy, 135
proliferative vitreo-retinopathy (PVR), 140
Prospective Evaluation of Radial Keratotomy (PERK), 11, 111
prosthetic eye, 141, 243
prosthetic lenses, 222
pseudostrabismus, 155
pterygium, 179–80
punctum, 23
pupils
  anatomy of, 26
  chromatic aberration of, 58–59
  dilation, 8–9, 44–47, 252–55
  dilator muscles, 27
  drug use and, 27, 252–55
  routine examination in, 37
  sphincter muscles, 27
purgatives, 2, 8

radial keratotomy (RK), 69, 113–20
  aftereffects of, 114–16
  common questions, 282
  described, 114
  origins of, 10–12, 114
  success of, 11–12, 117–20
  vision correction with, 116–17, 118–19, 120
Raphael, 6
reading glasses, 70, 286
reasonable and customary charges, 272
recession, 154–55
recurrent epithelial erosions, 120
recurrent erosion, of cornea, 165, 221–22
reflex tears, 172
refraction
  errors of. *see* refractive errors
  focusing light in, 59–65
  light sources in, 63
  testing, 190
refractive corneal keratectomy, 125–26

refractive errors, 38, 57–59
  and anisometropia, 58, 219–20, 228–29
  astigmatism. *see* astigmatism
  and eyeglass considerations, 69–71
  farsightedness. *see* farsightedness (hyperopia)
  nearsightedness. *see* nearsightedness (myopia)
refractive index, 60–61
refractive keratoplasty, 10–12, 121–22
refractive surgery, 109–28
  common questions, 282
  corneal. *see* corneal refractive surgery
  described, 109–11
  determining need for, 109–11
  with intraocular lenses, 112–13
  risks of, 111–12, 120
  surgeon selection for, 111–12
refractometry, 40–42
resection, 154
retina, 129–44
  age-related macular degeneration (ARMD), 130–34
  Amsler grid test for, 51
  anatomy of, 30–32
  arteries and veins of, 46–47
  central serous retinopathy, 137–38
  diabetic retinopathy, 134–36
  in dilated examination, 46, 68
  early awareness of, 4, 6
  HIV and, 140–41
  laser surgery for, 13
  macular holes, 136–37
  macular pucker, 137
  and physiology of sight, 129–30
  and pupil examination, 37
  retinal detachment and tears, 13, 45, 138–40
  and myopia, 68
  symptoms, 259–60
retinal edema, 135
retinal neovascularization, 135

retinal pigment epithelium (RPE) layer, 30
retinitis pigmentosa, 140–41
retinopathy of prematurity (ROP), 146–47
retinoscope, 41
retrolental fibroplasia (RLF), 146–47
rheumatoid arthritis, 23
rigid gas-permeable (RGP) lenses, 202, 215, 217, 219
  fitting and adaptation, 222–23
  orthokeratology and, 227–28
rods, 30, 51
Rohm and Haas Co., 216
Rome, ancient, 4
rubeosis, 43, 265
Ruiz, Richard, 122
Ruiz procedure, 127

Sato, 11, 114
Schachar Presbyopia Band, 286
Schirmer's tear test, 47–48
sclera
  anatomy of, 16–17, 19, 25
  early awareness of, 4
scleral buckle, 139
scleritis, 174, 175–76
seborrheic blepharitis, 159, 162
seborrheic dermatitis, 159
secondary carriers, insurance, 271
secondary cataracts, 74, 79, 91
secondary glaucoma, 99, 105, 120, 260
sedatives, 252
senile macular degeneration, 130–34
sickle cell disease, symptoms of, 46
slit lamp biomicroscope, 42, 45
slit lamp photographs, 50
"snake-eye" pupil, 100
Snellen test, 152
soft contact lenses, 201–2, 215–19
  bandage (BSCL), 221–22
  fitting and adaptation, 223–24
  infections and complications from, 224–27

Soviet Union, 10, 11
spectacles. *see* eyeglasses
sphincter muscles, 27
squamous cell carcinoma, 241
staph marginal ulcer, 226
staphylococcal blepharitis, 158–59, 161
staphyloma, 10, 134
staring eyelids, 237–38
state of indigency, 276
strabismus, 37, 66, 69, 148–55, 219
stroke, cerebral, 264
stroma
  anatomy of, 19, 20
  injuries to, 166
stromal infiltrates, 225–26
styes, 291
subconjunctival hemorrhage, 178–79
Sumerian empire, 1
superior, as term, 15
Supplemental Security Income (SSI), 273–76
surgery
  in ancient and classical periods, 1–4
  cataract. *see* cataract surgery
  corneal, 9–12, 126, 169–70, 178, 181–83
  for dry eyes, 173
  for epiphora, 174
  for glaucoma, 9, 101–6, 283
  in the Middle Ages, 4–6
  nineteenth century, 9
  ophthalmic plastic, 233–43
  for presbyopia, 286
  refractive. *see* refractive surgery
  removal of eye, 141, 243, 266
  retinal detachment, 139–40
  for strabismus, 154–55
  see also laser surgery
surgical iridectomy, 9
sweating, 8
synechiae, 98
syneresis, 45, 288

tarsorrhaphy, 173
tarsus, 158
tear enzymes, 19
tear (lacrimal) glands
  anatomy of, 22–23
  blocking of, 242–43
tears
  artificial, 23, 173, 242
  and dry eyes, 47–48, 172–73, 242
  excessive, 173–74, 241–43
tearsac infections, early treatment of, 1
temporal-arteritis, 260
temporal neurofibers, 30
temporomandibular joint (TMJ) headache, 290–91
thermokeratoplasty, 115, 126–27
thyroid disease, 237–38, 252
  exophthalmometry examination, 49
tinted contact lenses, 218–19
tonometry, 44, 105
toric contact lenses, 220
toric lenses, 58, 69
Touhy, Kevin, 216
toxoplasmosis, 133–34
trabecular meshwork, 26
  in glaucoma, 96
trabeculectomy, 103–4
trachoma, early treatment of, 1
tractional retinal detachment, 139–40
transplants, corneal, 9–12, 115, 121, 126, 169–70, 178, 181–83, 227
traumatic glaucoma, 99, 260
trial lens set, 42
trichiasis, 222
trifocal lenses, 40, 70–71
tumors, 260
  as cause of glaucoma, 99
  exophthalmometry examination, 49
  of the eyelids, 160, 240–41
  symptoms of, 46, 50

ulcerative keratitis, 202
ulcers, corneal, 170–72, 225
ultrasonography examination, 54
ultraviolet (UV) radiation
  cataracts from, 74
  epithelial burning from, 87, 263–64
  eyeglass filters, 200–201
uveitis, 105, 265–66
  as cause of glaucoma, 99

vascular insufficiency, symptoms of, 46
vasculitis, 260
venereal diseases, 7, 8
vergence, 59
versions, 37
Vesalius, Andreas, 6
vibgyor, 62
Vienna School, 8
viral conjunctivitis, 164
visible light, 60
vision examination, 38–40
visual cortex, 30, 129

visual field test, 48, 49, 95, 191
vitrectomy, 136, 137
vitreous (vitreous humor), 28
  detachment, 45
  in dilated examination, 45
vitreous cavity
  anatomy of, 18, 27–28
  early awareness of, 4
  floaters, 28, 43, 45, 288–89
vitreous hemorrhage, 260
vitritis, cataracts from, 74

wall eyes, 50
wandering eyes, 50
Wichterle, Otto, 216

YAG neodydium laser, 89–90, 91, 101, 104
YAG posterior capsulotomy, 79–80

zonular fibers, 28
zonules, 27

Additional copies of *YOUR VISION* may be ordered by sending a check for $19.95 (please add the following for postage and handling: $2.00 for the first copy, $1.00 for each additional copy) to:

MasterMedia Limited
17 East 89th Street
New York, NY 10128
(212) 260-5600
(800) 334-8232 *please use Mastercard or Visa on 1-800 orders*
(212) 546-7638 (fax)

OTHER MASTERMEDIA BOOKS

THE PREGNANCY AND MOTHERHOOD DIARY: Planning the First Year of Your Second Career, by Susan Schiffer Stautberg, is the first and only undated appointment diary that shows how to manage pregnancy and career. ($12.95 spiralbound)

CITIES OF OPPORTUNITY: Finding the Best Place to Work, Live and Prosper in the 1990's and Beyond, by Dr. John Tepper Marlin, explores the job and living options for the next decade and into the next century. This consumer guide and handbook, written by one of the world's experts on cities, selects and features forty-six American cities and metropolitan areas. ($13.95 paper, $24.95 cloth)

THE DOLLARS AND SENSE OF DIVORCE, by Dr. Judith Briles, is the first book to combine practical tips on overcoming the legal hurdles by planning finances before, during, and after divorce. ($10.95 paper)

OUT THE ORGANIZATION: New Career Opportunities for the 1990's, by Robert and Madeleine Swain, is written for the millions of Americans whose jobs are no longer safe, whose companies are not loyal, and who face futures of uncertainty. It gives advice on finding a new job or starting your own business. ($12.95 paper)

AGING PARENTS AND YOU: A Complete Handbook to Help You Help Your Elders Maintain a Healthy, Productive and Independent Life, by Eugenia Anderson-Ellis, is a complete guide to providing care to aging relatives. It gives practical advice and resources to the adults who are helping their elders lead productive and independent lives. Revised and updated. ($9.95 paper)

CRITICISM IN YOUR LIFE: How to Give It, How to Take It, How to Make It Work for You, by Dr. Deborah Bright, offers practical advice, in an upbeat, readable, and realistic fashion, for turning criticism into control. Charts and diagrams guide the reader into managing criticism from bosses, spouses, children, friends, neighbors, in-laws, and business relations. ($17.95 cloth)

BEYOND SUCCESS: How Volunteer Service Can Help You Begin Making a Life Instead of Just a Living, by John F. Raynolds III and Eleanor Raynolds, C.B.E., is a unique how-to book targeted at business and professional people considering volunteer work, senior citizens who wish to fill leisure time meaningfully, and students trying out various career options. The book is filled with interviews with celebrities, CEOs, and average citizens who talk about the benefits of service work. ($19.95 cloth)

MANAGING IT ALL: Time-Saving Ideas for Career, Family, Relationships, and Self, by Beverly Benz Treuille and Susan Schiffer Stautberg, is written for women who are juggling careers and families. Over two hundred career women (ranging from a TV anchorwoman to an investment banker) were interviewed. The book contains many humorous anecdotes on saving time and improving the quality of life for self and family. ($9.95 paper)

YOUR HEALTHY BODY, YOUR HEALTHY LIFE: How to Take Control of Your Medical Destiny, by Donald B. Louria, M.D., provides precise advice and strategies that will help you to live a long and healthy life. Learn also about nutrition, exercise, vitamins, and medication, as well as how to control risk factors for major diseases. Revised and updated. ($12.95 paper)

THE CONFIDENCE FACTOR: How Self-Esteem Can Change Your Life, by Dr. Judith Briles, is based on a nationwide survey of six thousand men and women. Briles explores why women so often feel a lack of self-confidence and have a poor opinion of themselves. She offers step-by-step advice on becoming the person you want to be. ($9.95 paper, $18.95 cloth)

THE SOLUTION TO POLLUTION: 101 Things You Can Do to Clean Up Your Environment, by Laurence Sombke, offers step-by-step techniques on how to conserve more energy, start a recycling center, choose biodegradable products, and even proceed with individual environmental cleanup projects. ($7.95 paper)

TAKING CONTROL OF YOUR LIFE: The Secrets of Successful Enterprising Women, by Gail Blanke and Kathleen Walas, is based on the authors' professional experience with Avon Products' Women of Enterprise Awards, given each year to outstanding women entrepreneurs. The authors offer a specific plan to help you gain control over your life, and include business tips and quizzes as well as beauty and lifestyle information. ($17.95 cloth)

SIDE-BY-SIDE STRATEGIES: How Two-Career Couples Can Thrive in the Nineties, by Jane Hershey Cuozzo and S. Diane Graham, describes how two-career couples can learn the difference between competing with a spouse and becoming a supportive power partner. Published in hardcover as *Power Partners*. ($10.95 paper, $19.95 cloth)

DARE TO CONFRONT! How to Intervene When Someone You Care About Has an Alcohol or Drug Problem, by Bob Wright and Deborah George Wright, shows the reader how to use the step-by-step methods of professional interventionists to motivate drug-dependent people to accept the help they need. ($17.95 cloth)

WORK WITH ME! How to Make the Most of Office Support Staff, by Betsy Lazary, shows you how to find, train, and nurture the "perfect" assistant and how to best utilize your support staff professionals. ($9.95 paper)

MANN FOR ALL SEASONS: Wit and Wisdom from The Washington Post's *Judy Mann,* by Judy Mann, shows the columnist at her best as she writes about women, families, and the impact and politics of the women's revolution. ($9.95 paper, $19.95 cloth)

THE SOLUTION TO POLLUTION IN THE WORKPLACE, by Laurence Sombke, Terry M. Robertson and Elliot M. Kaplan, supplies employees with everything they need to know about cleaning up their workspace, including recycling, using energy efficiently, conserving water and buying recycled products and nontoxic supplies. ($9.95 paper)

THE ENVIRONMENTAL GARDENER: The Solution to Pollution for Lawns and Gardens, by Laurence Sombke, focuses on what each of us can do to protect our endangered plant life. A practical sourcebook and shopping guide. ($8.95 paper)

THE LOYALTY FACTOR: Building Trust in Today's Workplace, by Carol Kinsey Goman, Ph.D., offers techniques for restoring commitment and loyalty in the workplace. ($9.95 paper)

DARE TO CHANGE YOUR JOB—AND YOUR LIFE, by Carole Kanchier, Ph.D., provides a look at career growth and development throughout the life cycle. ($9.95 paper)

MISS AMERICA: In Pursuit of the Crown, by Ann-Marie Bivans, is an authorized guidebook to the Pageant, containing eyewitness accounts, complete historical data, and a realistic look at the trials and triumphs of the potential Miss Americas. ($19.95 paper, $27.50 cloth)

POSITIVELY OUTRAGEOUS SERVICE: New and Easy Ways to Win Customers for Life, by T. Scott Gross, identifies what the consumers of the nineties really want and how businesses can develop effective marketing strategies to answer those needs. ($14.95 paper)

BREATHING SPACE: Living and Working at a Comfortable Pace in a Sped-Up Society, by Jeff Davidson, helps readers to handle information and activity overload, and gain greater control over their lives. ($10.95 paper)

TWENTYSOMETHING: Managing and Motivating Today's New Work Force, by Lawrence J. Bradford, Ph.D., and Claire Raines, M.A., examines the work orientation of the younger generation, offering managers in businesses of all kinds a practical guide to better understand and supervise their young employees. ($22.95 cloth)

REAL LIFE 101: The Graduate's Guide to Survival, by Susan Kleinman, supplies welcome advice to those facing "real life" for the first time, focusing on work, money, health, and how to deal with freedom and responsibility. ($9.95 paper)

BALANCING ACTS! Juggling Love, Work, Family, and Recreation, by Susan Schiffer Stautberg and Marcia L. Worthing, provides strategies to achieve a balanced life by reordering priorities and setting realistic goals. ($12.95 paper)

REAL BEAUTY . . . REAL WOMEN: A Handbook for Making the Best of Your Own Good Looks, by Kathleen Walas, International Beauty and Fashion Director of Avon Products, offers expert advice on beauty and fashion to women of all ages and ethnic backgrounds. ($19.50 paper)

THE LIVING HEART BRAND NAME SHOPPER'S GUIDE, by Michael E. DeBakey, M.D., Antonio M. Gotto, Jr., M.D., D.Phil., Lynne W. Scott, M.A., R.D./L.D., and John P. Foreyt, Ph.D., lists brand-name supermarket products that are low in fat, saturated fatty acids, and cholesterol. ($12.50 paper)

MANAGING YOUR CHILD'S DIABETES, by Robert Wood Johnson IV, Sale Johnson, Casey Johnson, and Susan Kleinman, brings help to families trying to understand diabetes and control its effects. ($10.95 paper)

STEP FORWARD: Sexual Harassment in the Workplace, What You Need to Know, by Susan L. Webb, presents the facts for identifying the tell-tale signs of sexual harassment on the job, and how to deal with it. ($9.95 paper)

A TEEN'S GUIDE TO BUSINESS: The Secrets to a Successful Enterprise, by Linda Menzies, Oren S. Jenkins, and Rickell R. Fisher, provides solid information about starting your own business or working for one. ($7.95 paper)

GLORIOUS ROOTS: Recipes for Healthy, Tasty Vegetables, by Laurence Sombke, celebrates the taste, texture, and versatility of root vegetables. Contains recipes for appetizers, soups, stews, and baked, boiled, and stir-fried dishes—even desserts. ($12.95 paper)

THE OUTDOOR WOMAN: A Handbook to Adventure, by Patricia Hubbard and Stan Wass, details the lives of adventurous outdoor women and offers their ideas on how you can incorporate exciting outdoor experiences into your life. ($14.95 paper)

FLIGHT PLAN FOR LIVING: The Art of Self-Encouragement, by Patrick O'Dooley, is a life guide organized like a pilot's flight checklist, which ensures you'll be flying "clear on top" throughout your life. ($17.95 cloth)

HOW TO GET WHAT YOU WANT FROM ALMOST ANYBODY, by T. Scott Gross, shows how to get great service, negotiate better prices, and always get what you pay for. ($9.95 paper)

TEAMBUILT: Making Teamwork Work, by Mark Sanborn, teaches business how to improve productivity, without increasing resources or expenses, by building teamwork among employers. ($19.95 cloth)

THE BIG APPLE BUSINESS AND PLEASURE GUIDE: 501 Ways to Work Smarter, Play Harder, and Live Better in New York City, by Muriel Siebert and Susan Kleinman, offers visitors and New Yorkers alike advice on how to do business in the city as well as how to enjoy its attractions. ($9.95 paper)